AIDS and the New Viruses

AIDS and the New Viruses

A. G. DALGLEISH

Clinical Research Centre, Division of Immunological Medicine, Harrow, UK

R. A. WEISS

Institute of Cancer Research, London, UK

ACADEMIC PRESS
Harcourt Brace Jovanovich, Publishers
London   San Diego   New York
Boston   Sydney   Tokyo   Toronto

This book is printed on acid-free paper.

Academic Press Limited
24–28 Oval Road
London NW1 7DX

United States edition published by
Academic Press Inc.
San Diego, CA 92101

British Library Cataloguing in Publication Data

AIDS and the new viruses.
1. Man. AIDS
I. Dalgleish, A. G.   II. Weiss, R.
616.9792

ISBN 0–12–200740–9

Typeset by Columns Design and Production Services Ltd, Caversham, Reading, Berks
Printed in Great Britain by Galliard (Printers) Ltd, Great Yarmouth, Norfolk

Contents

Contributors

Gordon L. Ada, Department of Immunology and Infectious Diseases, Johns Hopkins School of Hygiene and Public Health, Baltimore, MD 21205, USA

Angus G. Dalgleish, Retroviral Research Group, Division of Immunology, Clinical Research Centre, Watford Road, Harrow HA1 3UJ, UK

John A. Habeshaw, Retroviral Research Group, Clinical Research Centre, Watford Road, Harrow HA1 3UJ, UK

William A. Haseltine, Division of Human Retrovirology, Dana-Farber Cancer Institute, Harvard Medical School, Boston, MA 02115, USA

Robert W. Honess, Division of Virology, National Institute for Medical Research, The Ridgeway, Mill Hill, London NW7 1AA, UK

Meron Jacnya, Department of Medicine, Queen Elizabeth the Queen Mother Wing, St Mary's Hospital Medical School, London W2 1NY, UK

Peter Karayiannis, Department of Medicine, Queen Elizabeth the Queen Mother Wing, St Mary's Hospital Medical School, London W2 1NY, UK

Fabrizio Manca, Retroviral Research Group, Clinical Research Centre, Watford Road, Harrow HA1 3UJ, UK

Michelle E. D. Martin, Division of Virology, National Institute for Medical Research, The Ridgeway, Mill Hill, London NW7 1AA, UK

Jon Monjardino, Department of Medicine, Queen Elizabeth the Queen Mother Wing, St Mary's Hospital Medical School, London W2 1NY, UK

Andrew R. Moss, AIDS Epidemiology Group, Department of Epidemiology and International Health, San Francisco General Hospital, San Francisco, CA 94110, USA

John Saldanha, Department of Medicine, Queen Elizabeth the Queen Mother Wing, St Mary's Hospital Medical School, London W2 1NY, UK

Quentin J. Sattentau, Howard Hughes Medical Institute, College of Physicians and Surgeons, Columbia University, New York, NY 10032, USA

Thomas F. Schulz, Institute for Cancer Research, Fulham Road, London SW3 6BJ, UK

Howard C. Thomas, Department of Medicine, Queen Elizabeth the Queen Mother Wing, St Mary's Hospital Medical School, London W2 1NY, UK

Brian J. Thomson, Division of Virology, National Institute for Medical Research, The Ridgeway, Mill Hill, London NW7 1AA, UK

Johnathan Weber, Royal Postgraduate Medical School, Hammersmith Hospital, Ducane Road, London W12 0HS, UK

Robin Weiss, Institute of Cancer Research, Fulham Road, London SW3 6BJ, UK

David Wilks, Retroviral Research Group, Division of Immunology, Clinical Research Centre, Watford Road, Harrow HA1 3UJ, UK

Preface

A decade ago mankind seemed to be on the brink of conquering viral disease. Smallpox had finally been eradicated, safe and efficacious vaccines were becoming available for most of the serious childhood infections and there was a general air of confidence that virally induced cancers would similarly yield to preventive measures. The recognition of acquired immune deficiency syndrome (AIDS) in 1981 shattered our complacency. Nevertheless, there has been remarkable progress in our understanding of AIDS since the causative agent, human immuno-deficiency virus (HIV) was first isolated in 1983. The first six chapters in the volume chart the course of the AIDS epidemic, the molecular and cellular biology and pathology of HIV infection, and the prospects and problems in harnessing this knowledge for therapeutic and preventive means.

During the past decade other human viruses came to light for the first time, even though they may have an ancient provenance in human populations. The human T-cell leukaemia viruses (HTLV-I, HTLV-II) were discovered in 1980 and 1982 representing the first human retroviral pathogens, new human papilloma virus genomes (HPV-16, HPV-18) were identified in 1983 associated with cervical cancer, human herpes virus type 6 was recognised in 1987 and most recently in 1989, hepatitis C virus (HCV) has been identified among the non-A, non-B hepatitis infections. Some of these viruses (HTLV, HHV6) have been isolated by the classic method of propagation in culture, while others (HPV, HCV) were identified by molecular cloning.

The chapters contained in this volume were written to enable scientists and clinicians interested in human viral infection to obtain topical reviews that critically evaluate relevant data and concepts from the rapidly burgeoning literature. The chapters are contributed by leading investi-gators who have been enjoined to review a wide field without stifling their personal views. The subject matter is necessarily selective. We have, for example, omitted discussion of human papovaviruses or of the interesting animal lentiviruses related to HIV that have come to light since the discovery of HIV.

We are most grateful to the authors for their contributions and for ensuring that they are up to date including 1990 references. We thank Sue King at Academic Press for her understanding and persistence in producing this volume.

ANGUS G. DALGLEISH
ROBIN A. WEISS

1 | Clinical Epidemiology of AIDS and HIV Infection: What Do We Expect in the Second Decade of the Epidemic?

ANDREW R. MOSS

AIDS Epidemiology Group, Department of Epidemiology and International Health, San Francisco General Hospital, San Francisco, CA 94110, USA

1.1 INTRODUCTION

In 1989, eight years after the announcement of the first cases of AIDS in the USA, more than 130 000 cases have been reported world-wide. About 80 000 of these have been reported from the USA, 18 000 from Western Europe and 20 000 from Africa; however, the true extent of the epidemic in Africa is probably severely underreported. AIDS has now been seen in most countries of Europe, Africa and the Americas, and more recently in several Asian countries; thus in 1989 it has clearly taken its place as a world-wide epidemic. In broad terms, perhaps three to five million people world-wide are infected with HIV.

In 1989 AIDS is perhaps beginning to "mature" in the public perception, in that the reporting artifacts and illusions of the first years of the disease are fading and the probable long-term course of the epidemic is becoming clearer. From the point of view of epidemiology, some uncertainties about the general shape of the epidemic have been resolved over the past few years, two of which will be discussed here. The first is the question of which groups are at risk for HIV transmission, and in particular of the increasing importance of heterosexual transmission; the second is the question of the probable fate of the HIV-infected person.

1.2 CHANGE IN RISK GROUPS

1.2.1 Homosexual men

Although Western observers have become accustomed to thinking about AIDS as primarily a disease of homosexual men, this perspective is

AIDS AND THE NEW VIRUSES
ISBN 0–12–200740–9

rapidly becoming obsolete. In the USA in particular, new AIDS incidence has finally begun to reflect the changes in gay men's sexual behaviour that took place in the early 1980s. In San Francisco, where there are several studies of the historical pattern of HIV seroconversion in homosexual men, the seroconversion rate can be seen to have peaked at about 6000 new infections per year in 1982, or about 10–15% of the gay male population per year. The rate then declined sharply to 3–5% by 1984. Since then it has continued to fall, but more slowly, to about 1.0% per year in 1988. This rate represents perhaps 200 new infections in gay men in that year [1]. The majority of the gay men who have been infected in San Francisco were infected in the 1979–83 period, with a median date of infection of 1981. The AIDS incidence distribution which resulted from these infections has a much flatter and broader peak than the HIV seroconversion distribution because of the considerable individual variability in the "incubation period" from infection to AIDS. The incidence distribution appears to have flattened out at about 130–140 new cases a month in 1988 [2], and will probably soon begin to decline. Using the full pattern of seroconversion and incidence data for San Francisco, the average incubation period for clinical AIDS can be estimated to be 9.8 years from infection [1].

The same flattening of observed AIDS incidence rates in gay men has been reported in New York, with reported AIDS cases peaking in 1987 and perhaps declining slightly since then [3]; this has also occurred in Los Angeles. Thus in the three main American epidemic cities, AIDS cases in homosexual men seem to have peaked, and after a period of approximate stability, they can be expected to decline over the next few years. AIDS incidence in gay men has also flattened out in the UK [4].

In San Francisco the HIV seroconversion data can be shown to reflect the reported changes in gay mens' sexual behaviour — decreases in the number of sexual partners and in unprotected anal intercourse [5]. Similar changes in gay mens' sexual behaviour have been seen in many studies elsewhere in the USA and Europe. It is likely that AIDS incidence in gay men will decline world-wide over the next decade.

The gay male epidemic can be seen as a triumph for health education, with changes in risk behaviour seen quite soon after the original publicity about AIDS and the resulting changes in AIDS incidence showing up almost a decade later. In 1988 the shift in cases away from gay men to other risk groups was for the first time reflected in the Centers for Disease Control AIDS reporting data: the proportion of male cases in homosexual men fell from 70% in 1987 to 63% in 1988 [6]. In the Northeastern USA the proportion fell from 54% to 46%, so that for the first time homosexual men were not the majority of all new cases in that region. A similar shift has been reported in Western European countries by the WHO Collaborating Center on AIDS [7].

Estimating the size of the infected gay male population is difficult because homosexuality is hard to define and because the measured seropositivity rates may reflect men particularly at risk in the epidemic cities rather than gay men in general. The "official" US estimate, derived by the Centers for Disease Control (CDC) in 1987 and revised periodically, is 500 000–625 000 infected homosexual men [8], and is probably too high. A more realistic estimate based on back-calculation from observed progression rates to AIDS is 300 000–520 000 infected men [9]. Seroconversion rates are probably relatively low in most of the USA and most Western countries, so that the great proportion of all HIV infections in homosexual men have already happened. For homosexual men, with hundreds of thousands of infected men in Western countries but relatively low seroconversion rates, questions of prevention are now giving way to questions of early intervention and management of early HIV disease as the central issues in the medical politics of AIDS.

1.2.2 Intravenous drug users

As the proportion of new AIDS cases in homosexual men falls the proportion in the second major risk group, intravenous drug users (IVDUs), rises, both in the USA and in Western Europe. In the USA, IVDU cases rose from 14% of new male AIDS cases in 1987 to 20% in 1988 (from 34% to 41% in the Northeastern USA) [4]. In New York city, new AIDS cases in drug users overtook cases in homosexual men in 1987, and IVDU cases now predominate in three states — New York, New Jersey, Connecticut — and in Puerto Rico.

In Western Europe drug users comprised about 25% of all new AIDS cases in 1988, and in a broad belt across Southern and Central Europe, including much of Spain, the Mediterranean coast of France, Italy, central Switzerland and Yugoslavia, intravenous drug users are the bulk of all AIDS cases [7]. Recent data from Thailand also show a rapid rise in the proportion of HIV seropositive among the country's large IVDU population, raising the spectre of a rapid spread of HIV in other countries on the heroin trade routes such as Malaysia, Hong Kong and Pakistan. There is also concern about intravenous drug use in Brazil.

The gradual shift from gay men to intravenous drug users in the Western epidemic was amplified by the 1987 change in the CDC reporting definition of AIDS, which admitted presumptive diagnoses of opportunistic infections and wasting syndrome, both more prevalent in drug users than gay men. AIDS is still believed to be underreported in intravenous drug users as some clinical manifestations of HIV infection common in drug users are not regarded as reportable AIDS. The clinical spectrum of AIDS in drug users may differ considerably from that now familiar in gay men, and it is possible that in US cities such as New York, AIDS in drug users is underreported by as much as 50% [10].

The curve of reported AIDS cases in drug users is still rising rapidly in the USA. Sequential studies in New York and San Francisco suggest that the seropositivity rate in drug users rose rapidly from the late 1970s till about 1985, but has slowed since then, to perhaps 2-4% per year in both cities [11, 12]. It is therefore likely that new AIDS cases in drug users will continue to rise in the USA and Western Europe for at least the next few years, but will then turn down. Drug users may be the bulk of all new AIDS cases in the mid-1990s in both of these regions and in parts of Asia.

The implications of the shift in clinical case-load from gay men to drug users are considerable. First, the clinical pattern of AIDS in drug users is different from that in homosexual men. Recent studies suggest that HIV-infected drug users are susceptible to tuberculosis, bacterial pneumonia, and other manifestations of HIV, or other conditions exacerbated by HIV, so that clinical experience based on homosexual men may be inappropriate [11, 13]. Second, HIV-infected drug users are from a different social stratum than HIV-infected homosexual men. The latter are largely middle class, white, highly educated, and very responsive to education — hence the success of the "health education" approach. Drug users in the USA are largely black or hispanic and poor; in Europe they are from among the unemployed young. In both cases (and in Thailand and Brazil) intravenous drug users are from social strata which are out of contact with the health care system and unresponsive to health education; thus the prospects for long-term prevention in this risk group are less encouraging.

As with homosexual men, the number of infected intravenous drug users is hard to estimate. The same two US studies cited above estimate the number of infected drug users in the USA at 225 000 and 95 000–195 000, respectively in 1988 [8, 9]. Intravenous drug use is increasingly the dominant risk factor for HIV infection in Southern Europe, the Northeastern USA, and perhaps Asia. Although the size of the population at risk by intravenous drug use, and thus the size of the overall problem presented by HIV in this risk group, is limited, drug users are the source of most heterosexual AIDS in Western countries at present and of most paediatric AIDS. The drug-user epidemic is important beyond its size as the potential source of a heterosexual epidemic in Western, and perhaps other, countries.

1.2.3 Heterosexual transmission

Heterosexual transmission of HIV has been rare in Western countries, with 5% of total US cases and 8% of Western European cases currently attributed to heterosexual transmission, most of them in women. However, like the proportion of cases attributable to intravenous drug use, the proportion attributable to heterosexual transmission is rising in both regions.

In the USA about half of all heterosexual transmission cases are from an index case from a high risk country (most often Haiti): most of the rest are from an index case who is an intravenous drug user. Among women in the USA the proportion of all AIDS cases attributed to heterosexual transmission from a drug user or other high-risk partner rose from 15% before 1984 to 29% in 1988. There were an estimated 30 000 persons infected by heterosexual transmission in the USA in 1988 [8, 9].

The small number of heterosexual cases in Western countries is often contrasted with the very large number in Africa, where the sex ratio in reported AIDS cases is approximately 1:1 and where epidemic hetero-sexually transmitted AIDS is clearly a fact of life. HIV seroprevalence rates in general population groups — not "high risk" groups — were reported at between 10 and 20% in 1988 in studies in several African countries including Uganda, Rwanda, Zaire and Zambia [14] and may be increasing rapidly.

Much energy has been expended in trying to explain the difference between the African epidemic, a rapidly expanding general heterosexual epidemic, and what is perceived to be a very slowly growing, or even nonexistent, heterosexual epidemic in Western countries. Both biological and social explanations have been invoked, but at present the leading candidate is a "cofactor" explanation: the spread of HIV in Africa is promoted by ulcerative sexually transmitted diseases (STDs), which are thought to greatly increase the probability of HIV transmission. In one widely quoted study, ulcerative diseases were associated with a relative risk of seven in HIV transmission rates [15]. However, the cofactor explanation should probably be regarded with some caution until more data are available on the frequency of ulcerative STDs in African countries.

HIV transmission studies show a male–female transmission rate of 20–50% in most situations and the transmission rate seems to vary with progression of disease in the index case, and with prior STD exposure, and perhaps with frequency of anal sex. Transmission of HIV from women to men appears to be rare, at least in Western studies, but this phenomenon should also be treated with caution since very few female–to–male studies have been published, as most index cases are male in the Western epidemic. Cautiously, one might propose that heterosexual transmission has taken off slowly in Western countries because transmission probabilities are low, ulcerative STDs are rare, and the average number of sexual partners per year, at least in the preliminary studies done so far, is close to 1 [16].

While in Western countries as a whole heterosexual transmission is relatively rare in the general population, the apparent frequency of heterosexual infection in parts of the USA where intravenous drug use is widespread is beginning to cause alarm. Thus in 1988 studies of childbearing women in New York city, 1.25% of all newborn infants were HIV antibody positive at delivery, and 1.8% of all black infants [17]. Since about half of these infants are carrying maternal antibody only (the mother–child transmission probability is of the order of 50%), about 1% of all black infants in New York city were actually born HIV-infected in 1988. In parts of the city where intravenous drug use was widespread, the rate was higher. These rates would cause widespread alarm if they were found in any other social group. In addition, STD clinic and emergency room studies in inner cities are now finding HIV seroprevalence rates of 3–5% [18], not all of which can be explained by drug use. Although these studies are not yet producing direct measures of the seroconversion rate in high-risk heterosexuals, the seroprevalence rates are *already* sufficiently high in some cities in the Northeastern USA that public health officials should be considering intervention to stop sexual transmission.

In addition, after a generation of decline, syphilis is on the increase in the USA, with reported annual increases of 25% or more in 1984–87 in some Eastern cities [19]. Chancroid, also an ulcerative STD, has reappeared in the USA, primarily as a disease of the urban black poor and of migrant workers [20]. These ulcerative STDs are seen in the same inner-city black and hispanic and migrant labourer populations as HIV, thus there are no grounds for overconfidence about cofactors. Without significant intervention it is possible that a severe problem could materialize in these populations over the next decade.

As time passes, HIV, like most other infectious diseases, is increasingly revealing itself as a disease of poor people. In the USA, because the people at risk for heterosexual transmission are both poor and either black or hispanic, they are more like drug users than like gay men as targets of intervention: they are not easily accessible by health educators, and they are poorly served by the public health system. One canot but be pessimistic about the ability of the US public health system to deal with the problem of heterosexually transmitted HIV over the next decade. Comparable serological data is not yet available for those parts of

Southern Europe or Asia with major problems of HIV in drug users, and in these countries no newborn studies have yet been conducted; however, it is again likely that over the next decade there will be cause for concern.

1.3 PROGRESSION TO AIDS IN SEROPOSITIVE PERSONS

1.3.1 Progression rates over time

The new incidence rate of clinical AIDS in Western countries may be relatively stable over the 1990s, at least when compared with the rapid rise in the 1980s. However, there were already of the order of a million HIV-infected persons in the USA in 1989. There are probably several hundred thousand in other developed and developing countries in Europe, the Americas and Asia, and an unknown number, certainly in the millions, in Africa. Although it was once thought that only a fraction of those infected would become clinically sick, the current consensus is that HIV-infected persons must be expected to proceed to clinical AIDS [21, 22].

All prospective studies of HIV-infected homosexual men and others show a steadily rising probability of developing AIDS in the years following infection, with about half developing clinical AIDS by 10 years after infection in the one study followed this far [22]. Based on all the San Francisco data, the probabilities of developing AIDS in the first ten years after infection are zero, 1%, 2%, 4%, 6%, 7%, 8%, 8%, 7% and 7% respectively, and 50% will develop AIDS by 9.8 years after infection [1]. Most HIV-infected persons who have not been diagnosed with an AIDS manifestation show clinical or laboratory impairment predictive of AIDS by five years after infection, so that there is little doubt that in the absence of effective treatment, most will eventually progress to AIDS. Preliminary studies suggest that progression rates in haemophiliacs and intravenous drug users are similar to those in homosexual men.

As a result of the prospective studies, the consensus about AIDS and HIV has changed. "AIDS" is increasingly thought of not as an abrupt, acute illness characterized by an estimated survival time of months from diagnosis [23], but as the late stage in a long-term chronic "HIV disease" whose course may run 10 years or more. Clinical and laboratory markers measured during the long course of infection can thus be used to anticipate clinical AIDS and to improve the delivery of prophylactic or acute treatment.

1.3.2   Predictors of progression

Among the clinical predictors used to predict AIDS, persistent lymphadenopathy, which was originally thought to predict imminent disease, is
now thought to be associated with seroconversion and not a predictor of
progression. Currently used clinical predictors in studies of homosexual
men are herpes zoster, usually diagnosed at 2–7 years from infection,
thrush and/or hairy leukoplakia, probably usually diagnosed slightly later
in infection, and lymphoma-like "constitutional symptoms" (persistent
night sweats, fevers, weight loss or diarrhoea), usually diagnosed
relatively late in infection and thus good predictors of imminent AIDS
[20]. Two-year progression rates to AIDS for HIV-infected men with
lymphadenopathy, shingles, thrush, hairy leukoplakia and constitutional
symptoms were 22, 25, 39, 42 and 100% respectively in one study,
compared with a 16% progression rate over two years in men with no
symptoms [22].

Laboratory markers used to predict AIDS in HIV seropositive persons
include CD4 lymphocyte count, presence of the HIV p24 core antigen,
serum β-2 microglobulin, and serum neopterin [24]. CD4 lymphocyte
counts fall by 60–100 mm^3 per year in HIV infected homosexual men
from a normal value of 800–900 mm^3, and asymptomatic men with less
than 200 mm^3 can be shown to have a three-year probability of
progression to AIDS of more than 80%. Similarly, men with detectable
p24 antigen, or with serum β-2 microglobulin greater than 5.0 mg/l, can
be shown to have an expected progression rate to AIDS of more than
70% over three years. These and other markers can be combined to give
a very good multivariate prediction of the imminence of AIDS in HIV-
infected homosexual men, and they are also being explored in studies of
HIV-infected intravenous drug users and haemophiliacs. The same
markers can be shown to reflect the antiviral activity of aziodothymidine
(AZT) in clinical trials [25].

Finally, improved treatment for AIDS is now being extended to the
population of seropositive people at high risk for clinical disease. Both
AZT and aerosolized pentamidine are available for symptomatic persons
or those with CD4 count less than 200 mm^3, and AZT (and probably
soon pentamidine) is under investigation in persons who are early in the
course of infection. The effect of these therapies on survival after an
AIDS diagnosis has already been considerable: survival after diagnosis
with an opportunistic infection in San Francisco has probably doubled
from the 9 months reported in the early years and it continues to rise [23,
26]. As these and other therapies become available early in the course of
HIV infection, the current 10 or 12 year life span of an HIV-infected

person will increase and AIDS will increasingly be seen as a long-term chronic condition rather than as an acute disease.

1.4 PROSPECT FOR THE 1990s

It seems likely that Western countries are approaching a period of rough stability in their AIDS case-loads in the 1990s, as cases in homosexual men go down and those in drug users and heterosexuals go up. It is likely however that both the clinical and service-provision pictures will shift considerably, reflecting the changing populations developing disease, and in particular reflecting the shift towards the urban poor as the main group at risk. Whether this period of stability in the 1990s is followed by a second rapid increase in the AIDS case-load in the following decade probably depends on whether an effective prevention strategy can be developed for the long-term problem of heterosexual transmission.

In the interim, as more infected persons come to be identified and as the therapeutic picture improves, we will increasingly be faced with the problem of long-term management of seropositive persons, many of whom will be infected but well (and many of whom will be infectious) for a decade or more. In the likely absence of either magic-bullet therapies or vaccines in the next decade, the main problem in AIDS may well be getting Western, as well as Third World, societies to face up to the management of HIV disease in large numbers of chronically infected persons among the urban poor.

REFERENCES

1. Bachetti, P. and Moss, A.R. (1989). Incubation period of AIDS in San Francisco. *Nature, Lond.* **338**, 251–253.
2. *AIDS Monthly Surveillance Report*. San Francisco, Department of Public Health, May 1989.
3. Statement of Dr S.C. Joseph, Health Commissioner. New York City Department of Health, May 1988.
4. AIDS Update (1989). *Br. Med. J.* **298**, 1057.
5. Coates, T.J., Stall, R.D. and Hoff, C. (1988). Changes in sexual behavior of homosexual and bisexual men since the beginning of the AIDS epidemic. US Congress, Office of Technology Assessment.
6. CDC (1989). Update: Acquired Immunodeficiency syndrome in the United States. *MMWR* **38**, 229–236.
7. AIDS Surveillance in Europe: Quarterly Report No. 19, September 1988. WHO Collaborating Center on Aids, Paris, 1988.
8. CDC (1988). Human Immunodeficiency Virus infection in the United States: A review of current knowledge. *MMWR* **36**, No. S–6, p. 15.

9. Osmond, D.H. and Moss, A.R. (1989). The prevalence of HIV infection in the United States: A reappraisal of the Public Health Service estimate. *AIDS Clin. Rev.*, 1–17.

10. Stoneburner, R., Laussucq, S., Benezra, D. *et al.* (1988). Increasing pneumonia mortality in NYC 1980–86. Evidence for a larger spectrum of HIV-related disease in intravenous drug users. *IVth International Conference on AIDS*, Stockholm, June 1988 (Abstract 7133).

11. Des Jarlais, D., Sotheran, J., Stoneburner, R. *et al.* (1988). HIV-1 is associated with fatal infectious disease other than AIDS in intravenous drug users. *IVth International Conference on AIDS*, Stockholm, June 1988 (Abstract 4219).

12. Moss, A.R., Chaisson, R., Osmond, D., Bacchetti, P. and Meakin, R. (1988). Control of HIV infection in San Francisco intravenous drug users. *IVth International Conference on AIDS*, Stockholm, June 1988 (Abstract 8630).

13. Selwyn, P.A., Shoenbaum, E.E., Harter, D. *et al.* (1988). AIDS and HIV related mortality in intravenous drug users. *IVth International Conference on AIDS*, Stockholm, June 1988 (Abstract 4526).

14. N'Galy, B. and Ryder, R.W. (1988). Epidemiology of HIV infection in Africa. *J. AIDS* **1**, 551–558.

15. Simonsen, J.N., Cameron, D.W., Gakinya, M.N. *et al.* (1988). Human immunodeficiency virus infection among men with sexually transmitted diseases. *New Engl. J. Med.* **319**, 274–278.

16. Skegg, D.C.G. (1989). Heterosexually acquired HIV infection. *Br. Med. J.* **298**, 401–402.

17. Novick, L.F., Berns, D., Stricof, R., Stevens, R., Pass, K. and Wethers, J. (1989). HIV seroprevalence in newborns in New York State. *J. Am. Med. Assoc.* **261**, 1745–1750.

18. Quinn, T.C., Glasser, D.S., Cannon, R.O. *et al.* (1988). Human immunodeficiency virus infection among patients attending clinics for sexually transmitted diseases. *New Engl. J. Med.* **318**, 197–202.

19. CDC (1988). Relationship of syphilis to drug use and prostitution. *MMWR* **37**, 755–758.

20. Mindel, A. (1989). Chancroid. *Br. Med. J.* **298**, 64–65.

21. Lifson, A.R., Rutherford, G.W. and Jaffe, H.W. (1988). The natural history of infection with HIV. *J. Infect. Dis.* **158**, 1360–1367.

22. Moss, A.R. and Bacchetti, P. (1989). Natural history of HIV infection. *AIDS* **3**, 55–61.

23. Bacchetti, P., Osmond, D.H., Chaisson, R. *et al.* (1988). Survival patterns of the first 500 patients with AIDS in San Francisco. *J. Infect. Dis.* **157**, 1044–1047.

24. Moss, A.R. (1988). Predicting who will progress to AIDS: at least four laboratory predictors available. *Br. Med. J.* **297**, 1067–1068.

25. Jacobson, M.A., Abrams, D.I., Volberding, P. *et al.* (1989). Serum Beta-2 microglobulin decreases in AIDS and ARC patients treated with azidothymidine. *J. Infect. Dis.* **159**, 1029–1036.

26. San Francisco Department of Public Health (1988). Survival following diagnosis of AIDS-related opportunistic infection. *San Francisco Epidemiol. Bull.* **4** (12), 49–50.

2 | Molecular Biology of HIV-1

WILLIAM A. HASELTINE

Dana-Farber Cancer Institute, Harvard Medical School, Boston, MA 02115, USA

2.1 INTRODUCTION

The human immunodeficiency virus type 1 (HIV-1) may establish three types of infection — active, controlled and silent (Fig. 2.1). During active infection abundant virus can be detected in most body fluids. Prolonged active replication is correlated with progressive degenerative disease of the immune, central nervous and other organ systems. Only very small amounts of virus are found during the state of controlled infection but very high antibodies to a broad array of viral proteins are present — indicative of low level chronic virus production. No virus particles or antiviral antibodies can be detected in silent infections but viral DNA can be detected using gene amplification techniques. Live virus can be isolated from some people who harbour silent infections.

Molecular studies of HIV-1 have progressed to the point where it is now possible to begin to understand the complexity of the interactions of HIV-1 with the host in terms of the structure and function of the virus-specified proteins.

2.2 THE VIRUS PARTICLE AND LIFE-CYCLE

The virus particle comprises an inner core that contains viral RNA and enzymes required for early steps of replication (Fig. 2.2). The virus is surrounded by a lipid membrane. A matrix protein (p17) lines the inner surface of the membrane. The outer surface of the particle comprises an envelope protein organized into spikes. This protein is embedded in the lipid membrane. Viral proteins are encoded by three genes that, respectively, encode the capsid protein, the replicative enzymes, and the envelope protein. The capsid proteins are made as a single polypeptide chain and cleaved late in virus maturation by a viral protease. The

AIDS AND THE NEW VIRUSES
ISBN 0–12–200740–9

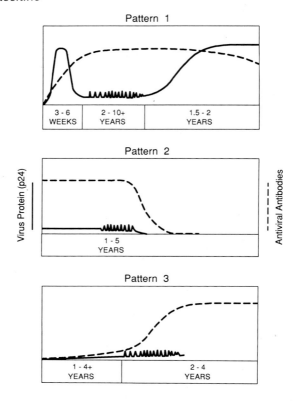

Fig. 2.1 Patterns of HIV-1 replication in infected people. The solid line represents viral particles in serum. The dashed line represents antiviral antibodies.

replicative enzymes are made from an elongated capsid polypeptide precursor, the result of a shift in the translation reading frame at a specific site in the region of overlap between the capsid and replicative genes, an event that occurs at a frequency of 1 in 20 [1]. The full length RNA transcript of the viral DNA serves as the messenger RNA for the capsid and replicative genes.

The envelope protein is made as a single large polypeptide. The protein is very heavily modified by addition of complex carbohydrates via the action of cellular enzymes [2, 3]. The envelope protein is transported to the cell surface where it is cleaved by cellular enzymes. The amino-terminal portion of the protein is located entirely exterior to the cell membrane and is non-covalently associated with the carboxy terminus that is anchored to the viral membrane. The association of the envelope protein with the core occurs as the virus buds from the cell surface.

(a)

Virion Proteins

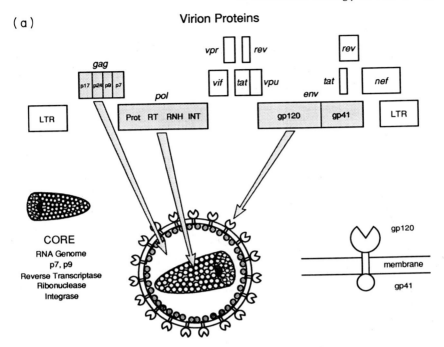

Fig. 2.2 (a) A schematic representation of the HIV-1 genome and viral particle. The shaded regions represent genes for proteins which are known to comprise the virus particle. The unshaded regions represent regulatory regions or regulatory genes. (b) (see over) A partial list of messenger DNA specified by HIV-1. TAR is the *tat* responsive sequence, CAR is a sequence necessary for *rev*. CRS suppresses structural protein expression in the absence of *rev*. The mRNAs below line accumulate in the absence of *rev*. Accumulation of mRNAs above the line requires the presence action of *rev*.

There are two phases to HIV replication, establishment, and expression (Fig. 2.3). Infection is established when the virus particle binds to the cell surface and enters via membrane-to-membrane fusion [4]. On entry, the single-stranded viral RNA is converted to double-stranded DNA by the conservative action of two enzymes packaged within the capsid, the polymerase and the ribonuclease [5]. It is likely the capsid proteins play some role in this stage of viral replication as well. The DNA migrates to the nucleus and, with the cooperation of a viral protein that is also packaged in the capsid, *gag* — the integrase protein — is inserted into the cellular DNA [5]. Once part of the cellular DNA, the viral genetic information remains in the cell as long as the cell survives. HIV infects cells that are long-lived. Some of these cells are not killed by infection and in others infection is silent. *Life-long persistent infection*

(b)

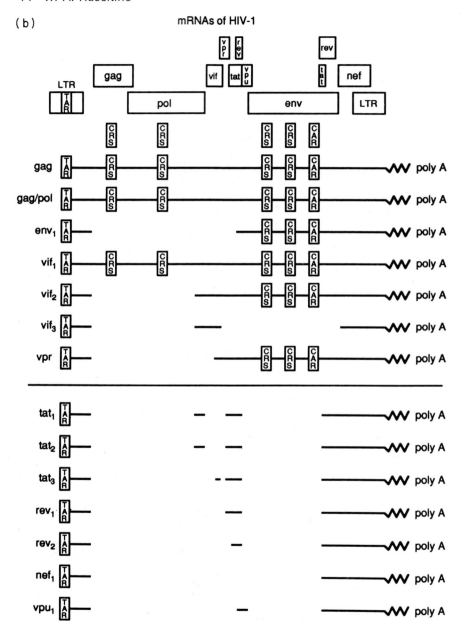

Fig. 2.2 *Continued*

HIV-1 Life-cycle

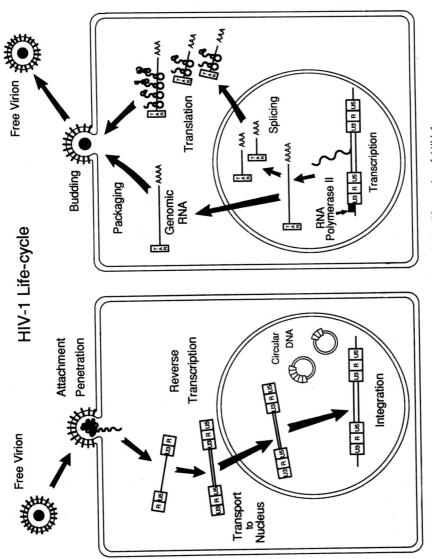

Fig. 2.3 A schematic representation of the life-cycle of HIV-1.

with HIV is a consequence of the life-cycle of the virus, a virus that becomes part of the DNA of the cells that it infects.

Expression of virus begins with formation of viral RNA copies of the viral DNA carried about by host cell RNA polymerases. Cellular enzymes process the initial RNA transcript, yielding a complex pattern of subfragments of the initial transcript that serve as messenger RNA for some of the viral proteins. The full-length transcript is incorporated into newly formed virus particles and serves as genetic information for the next generation of virus — messenger RNAs direct synthesis of the viral proteins that are assembled into the mature virus particle (for a review, see [6]). *In many cells, replication of the virus can occur without cell death. Chronic production of low levels of virus in patients is the result of non-cytopathic infection of some tissues.*

2.3   CONTROLLED REPLICATION

The most surprising discovery coming from the molecular analysis of HIV-1 is the existence of an elaborate set of regulatory genes that in the first instance determine whether or not virus is made, and if virus is made, control the level of virus production. The existence of these genes was not anticipated because they are not present in retroviruses that have been studied previously. The existence of such genes was foreshadowed only by the discovery of a regulatory gene in the second class of pathogenic human retroviruses, the human T cell leukaemia virus, HTLV-1, in 1984 [7].

2.4   THE LONG TERMINAL REPEAT

The long terminal repeat (LTR) flanks the proviral DNA and contains signals that govern transcriptional initiation and termination. The LTR contains numerous sites that have been recognized as binding factors that facilitate RNA initiation, including the TATAA sequence, CAAT sequence and sequences which bind SP-1 [8–10] (Fig. 2.4). The LTR contains two sequences which recognize proteins that bind to DNA when T cells are activated — the NK $\varkappa$ B and NFAT-1 sites [11, 12]. These two sequences play an important role in the virus life-cycle. In resting T cells very little, if any, RNA is made. When T cells are activated by specific or non-specific stimuli, viral RNA is made and virus replication begins. The ability of the virus to lie dormant in circulating T cells can be attributed, at least in part, to the dependence of NF $\varkappa$ B and NFAT-1 for viral transcription.

The LTR also contains sequences which suppress initiation called the negative regulatory element (NRE) [13, 14]. Deletion of this sequence yields virus which produce five times as much virus in T cell lines and 30 times as much virus in monocyte cell lines [15]. The NRE also contains sequences that recognize cellular proteins.

The existence of the *cis*-acting negative sequence may help to explain the very low rate of virus replication, particularly in monocytes and macrophages.

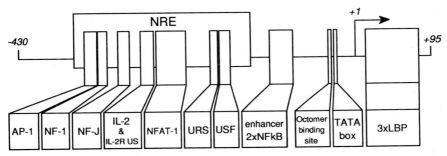

Fig. 2.4 A schematic representation of the HIV-1 LTR illustrating consensus binding sites for cellular nuclear proteins involved in transcription initiation.

2.5 POSITIVE REGULATION

2.5.1 Transactivator (*tat*)

There are two types of regulatory genes that accelerate virus replication. The *trans*-activator gene (*tat*) is a positive feedback regulator that increases the rate of its own synthesis and the synthesis of all viral proteins [16] (Fig. 2.5(a)). It is an essential gene because *tat*-negative mutants do not replicate [17, 18].

There are two components to most genetic regulatory pathways: a diffusible effector molecule — often a protein — and a *cis*-acting responsive element — often the nucleic-acid sequence. In the case of the *tat* regulatory pathway, the effector is an 86 amino acid long protein [19, 20]. The protein is located in the nucleus and nucleolus of infected cells [21, 22]. The responsive element is a short segment of nucleic acid called the *trans*-activating responsive region (TAR) located between +1 and +45 of the genome, +1 being the initial nucleotide of the viral RNA [20, 23–25]. The TAR sequence can assume a stable double-stem loop configuration [26, 27]. Current evidence indicates that the critical

(a)

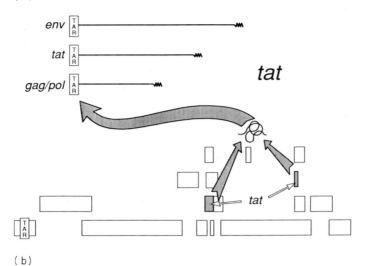

(b)

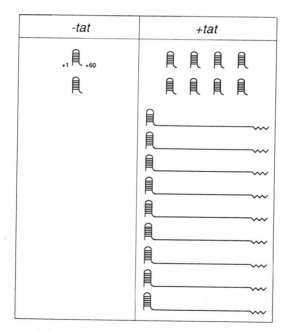

Fig. 2.5   (a) A schematic representation highlighting the two coding exons of *tat*, and illustrating the action of *tat* in *trans* on mRNAs which contain TAR. (b) A representation of the HIV-1 RNA species which accumulate in the absence or presence of *tat*.

sequences of TAR are located at the tip of the first loop [28]. Current evidence also indicates that the TAR sequence prevents efficient use of messenger RNA in the absence of the *tat* protein. In the presence of the *tat* protein, such inhibition is abrogated and RNA initiated by the TAR sequence directs protein synthesis with extraordinary efficiency [29–31]. There are several reports that *tat* protein binds directly to TAR RNA (J. Karn, C.A. Rosen and F. Wong-Staal, personal communications).

The *tat* product may, under appropriate conditions, accelerate the production of viral proteins by several thousand-fold. The synthesis of all viral proteins, both those that comprise the virion and the regulatory proteins themselves, are affected by *tat* because all viral messenger RNAs contain the TAR sequence at the 5′ end [23]. In the absence of *tat* fragments of the 5′ viral RNA, nucleotides 1–60, accumulate (Fig. 2.5(b)). Three possible explanations have been advanced to explain this observation:

(1) *tat* overcomes transcription attenuation.
(2) *tat* prevents nuclease degradation of viral RNA.
(3) *tat* permits rapid exit of viral RNA from the nucleus wherein nucleases degrade the RNA to a 60 nucleotide RNA-resistant fragment.

2.6 AN UNUSUAL GENETIC SWITCH — (*rev*)

The regulator of virion protein expression, *rev*, is a gene that positively regulates expression of virion proteins, but negatively regulates the expression of regulatory genes [32–34] (Fig. 2.6(a)). There are two *cis*-acting sequences that are part of the *rev* regulatory pathways. One of these *cis*-acting sequences acts to prevent RNA expression. This element is called the *cis*-acting repression sequence (CRS) [29]. Multiple CRS elements exist in the viral coding sequences. There is at least one CRS element in the capsid coding sequences, one in the sequences that encode the replicative genes, and at least two in the envelope glycoprotein. The genes that encode the regulatory proteins are devoid of CRS sequences. When present in the RNA, the CRS sequences prevent the message from being used as a substrate for protein synthesis. It is suspected that these sequences specify retention of the viral RNA in a nuclear compartment that contains splicing and powerful degradative activities.

A sequence exists in the envelope gene that is required for *rev* protein-dependent relief of CRS expression, the *cis*-acting antirepression sequences (CAR) also called *rev* repressive element (RRE) [35–37]. The CAR element is responsive to the *rev* protein. The interaction between

(a)

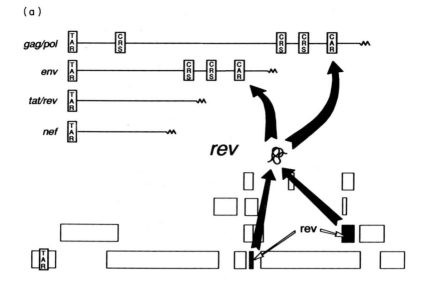

(b)

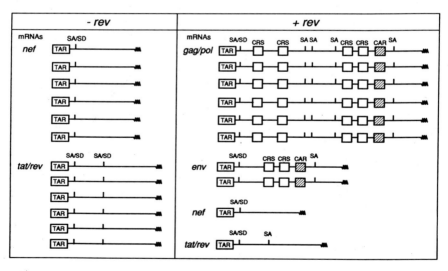

Fig. 2.6 (a) A schematic representation of *rev* action highlights the two coding exons of *rev* and the location of CAR and CRS sequences in HIV-1 mRNAs. (b) A summary of HIV-1 mRNA accumulation in the absence and presence of *rev*.

the *rev* product and the CAR sequence overrides the repressive effects of CRS sequences and permits use of messenger RNAs for protein synthesis. There is evidence that the interaction between the CAR and *rev* product permits transport of the RNA that contains CRS from the subnuclear compartment that contains splicing and degradative enzymes to a compartment in which splicing can no longer occur and from which the RNA may gain access to the translational machinery.

In the absence of the *rev* protein, RNA species accumulate that have had the viral structural genes removed by splicing [33, 38] (Figs 2.2(b), 2.6(b)). Removal of the virus structural genes by splicing also removes the CRS sequences. These small RNAs are those that encode the regulatory proteins. In the presence of the *rev* protein, full-length RNAs and RNA that encodes the *env* proteins accumulate, and the concentration of messenger RNAs that specify regulatory proteins decreases.

2.6   NEGATIVE REGULATION

2.6.1   Negative regulation factor (*nef*)

The effector of the negative regulatory factor (*nef*) pathway is a protein that is located in the cytoplasm and retards virus replication [39–42] (Fig. 2.7). The 27-kD protein is specified by a messenger RNA that has all of the sequences of the capsid, replicative, and envelope genes removed by splicing [43]. Mutants defective for *nef* replicate more rapidly than *nef*$^+$ virus.

The *nef* protein has interesting biochemical properties. One form of the protein contains a fatty acid, myristic acid, at the amino terminus, suggesting that this form of the protein is embedded in the inner surface of the cell membrane [44]. The *nef* protein is reported to bind GTP and have a GTPase activity [45]. The protein is also reported to be a protein kinase capable of autophosphorylation and is a substrate of protein kinase C [45]. The *nef* protein may act as an analogue of signal-transducing proteins by modifying cellular proteins that regulate transcription initiation.

2.7   VIRION INFECTIVITY FACTOR — (*vif*)

HIV-1 also specifies a protein that increases the infectivity of the virus particle. The gene that specifies this protein is called the virion infectivity gene (*vif*) [46, 47]. The protein is present in the cytoplasm of infected

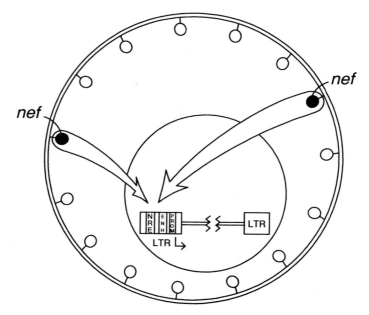

Fig. 2.7 A schematic representation of *nef* action illustrating the negative effect of *nef* on viral replication. The presumed role of *nef* in nuclear function is speculative.

cells and can also be found outside the cells [47]. Virus defective for this function have a normal appearance and bind with normal efficiency to the surface of susceptible cells. Current evidence indicates that the *vif* protein increases the efficiency of the step that occurs after virus attachment, but before the viral DNA is integrated in the host cell DNA [44, 48].

It is likely that efficient cell-to-cell and possibly the efficiency of person-to-person spread of HIV-1 is partly a consequence of the increased infectivity of cell-free viruses attributable to the vif *product.*

2.8   VIRAL PROTEIN U — (*vpu*)

The *vpu* protein facilitates assembly and budding of viral particles. Five to ten times more virus is released from T cells infected with vpu^+ as compared to isogenic vpu^- virus [49–51] (Fig. 2.8). Paradoxically, the vpu^- virus are more rapidly lethal to CD4+ T cells as judged by syncytia formation and single cell killing. Evidently, cell-associated viral protein, except probably *env* protein on the surface of the CD4+ T cell, is required for cytopathic effect.

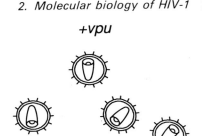

-*vpu*   +*vpu*

Fig. 2.8   A schematic diagram illustrating the effect of *vpu* on viral particle output.

The combined action of the two viral genes, *vif* and *vpu*, results in production of large amounts of highly infectious virus — facilitating cell-to-cell and person-to-person transmission.

2.9   VIRAL PROTEIN R — (*vpr*)

HIV-1 specifies a second transactivator, the product of *vpr*. This gene specifies a 15-kD protein (E.A. Cohen, E. Terwilliger and W.A. Haseltine, unpublished observations). The protein acts in *trans* to accelerate the rate of viral protein production. The product of *vpr* is capable of stimulating expression of homologous and of heterologous genes in *trans* and may alter some cell functions (E.A. Cohen, E. Terwilliger and W.A. Haseltine, unpublished observations). It is curious that, like *vpu* and *nef*, *vpr* is defective in many cultured HIV-1 isolates.

2.10   A REGULATORY NETWORK

The genes of HIV that affect the rate of viral replication also regulate one another. A diagram of some of the interactions among these regulatory proteins is depicted in Fig. 2.9.

Consider the interactions of separate components of this regulatory network. The *tat* product positively regulates *rev* and itself. The *rev* product negatively regulates *tat* and itself as it suppresses the accumulation of the spliced RNAs from which *tat* and *rev* are made. The result should be a steady-state level of both proteins. Similar positive regulation

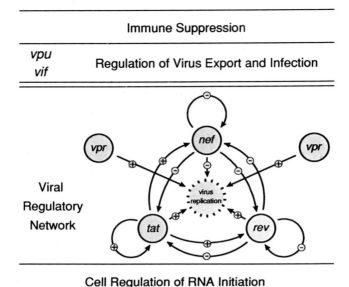

Immune Suppression

vpu
vif   Regulation of Virus Export and Infection

Viral
Regulatory
Network

Cell Regulation of RNA Initiation

Fig. 2.9 A schematic diagram of levels of HIV-1 regulation. Interactions among the HIV-1 viral regulatory genes are illustrated.

of *nef* by *tat* and negative regulation of *tat* by *nef* should result in steady-state levels of both proteins. Such regulation should permit controlled replication of the virus. The actual level of viral replication will be dependent on the intracellular conditions that determine the relative levels of each protein and the relative frequency of specific splicing events.

The consequences of interactions of the *rev* and *nef* pathways are different. The *rev* product suppresses the production of the *nef* gene and itself by preventing accumulation of spliced forms of RNA from which both proteins are made. The *nef* product suppresses the synthesis of all viral RNAs by decreasing the rate of RNA initiation. The *rev–nef* interaction may provide an all-or-none switch for virus replication. If *nef* protein accumulates first, then virus replication may be suppressed for prolonged periods. If *rev* accumulates first, abundant or controlled replication may occur. Changes in intracellular conditions that affect relative *nef* and *rev* activities may either induce productive replication or permit productively infected cells to turn off replication and enter a latent state.

The *cis-* and *trans-*acting regulatory elements of RNA are sufficient to account for the complexity of virus–virus and virus–cell interactions that have been observed. Silent infections may be interpreted as establishment of latent infections via the action of the negative regulatory genes and infection of resting cell populations. Controlled replication can be interpreted in terms of steady-state levels of positive and negative regulatory proteins that, in turn, lead to controlled levels of viral synthesis. Prolific replication can be interpreted as either being due to perturbations of the regulatory network or to an increase in infections of populations of cells that can lead to high-level productive infection.

The regulatory network may also help to account for the switch from silent to controlled infections and from controlled replication to silent infection.

2.11 A MODEL FOR PROGRESSIVE DISEASE

Progressive disease appears to be a consequence of the gradual rise in virus replication rate after a prolonged period of controlled replication. A dynamic model based on known properties of HIV-1 may account for the slow but inexorable switch from controlled to prolific replication (Fig. 2.10). One cell type in which prolific replication is known to occur is the activated CD4+ T lymphocyte. Infection of such cells results in the rapid production of prodigious quantities of virus [52–54]. However, infection of resting CD4+ T lymphocytes results in latent infection. At any time, the fraction of CD4+ lymphocytes actually replicating in the blood is very small — approximately one in 10 000 [55]. Consequently, most infections of this population result in latent infection. Over time, the low level of virus produced by infected monocytes and other cell types should eventually increase the fraction of CD4+ cells that are latently infected. Over a prolonged period, the probability that a latently infected T cell will be activated at random will increase. Activation of the latently infected T cells should result in a large burst of virus release. This process should be autocatalytic. The result should eventually be a switch from a state of controlled replication to a state of continued high-level virus production.

2.12 GENOMIC VARIABILITY

Independent HIV isolates vary from one another by 20–25% of the nucleic acid sequence. Similar variation is noted in predicted amino acid

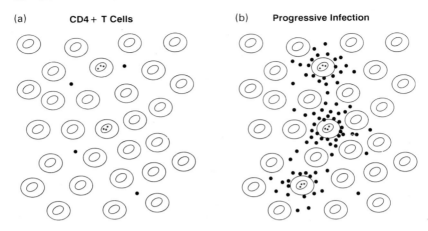

(a)   CD4+ T Cells

(b)   Progressive Infection

Fig. 2.10 A model for HIV-1 induced progressive disease. (a) Early in infection only a few CD4+ T cells harbour latent virus. (b) Later, more CD4+ T cells harbour latent virus, increasing the likelihood that an infected T cell will be activated to produce more virus — a self-accelerating process.

sequences. What is the source of such variation and what are the implications of variations for pathogenesis and transmission of the virus?

The changes from one HIV strain to another occur by sequential mutation — changes in single bases, as well as small deletions and duplications. Such mutations are primarily introduced during replication. Replication of all retroviruses, including HIV, involves three separate conversions of nucleic acid. The virus polymerase converts the genomic viral RNA to DNA and the resultant RNA/DNA hybrid to a double-stranded DNA form. The nascent viral genome is made by copying the viral DNA by the cellular RNA polymerase. All three conversion steps introduce errors. The viral polymerase and cellular RNA polymerases do not have the ability to remove incorrectly base-paired nucleotides once incorporated. Moreover, viral DNA is made in the cytoplasm whereas most of the cellular enzymes that recognize mismatched nucleotides, small deletions, or duplications are present in the nucleus. No enzymatic means is known for correction of RNA that is incorrectly copied from DNA.

The error frequency during replication may be expressed as:

$$E = (2 \times [\text{error frequency of viral polymerase}] \\ + [\text{error frequency of RNA polymerase}] \\ + [\text{error frequency of cellular RNA replication}]) \\ \times N$$

The last term of this equation reflects the error frequency of cellular DNA replication, where N represents the number of divisions of a cell that harbours a latent provirus. Under most conditions, this term will be very small because cellular DNA replication has an error frequency of the order of one mistake per billion nucleotides copied.

The error frequency for a single round of replication from a DNA to DNA form of an avian leukosis virus has been determined to be approximately one point mutation per 10 000 nucleotides and one deletion or duplication per 10 000 nucleotides. *This mutation rate means that on average there is one point mutation and one deletion or duplication introduced per viral genome per round of replication.* Variation of retroviruses is an inevitable consequence of replication — the more rounds of replication, the more mutation. The rapid rate of variation in HIV isolates therefore represents numerous rounds of replication that intervene between isolates.

It is likely that most mutants will result in non-viable virus. Attempts to clone infectious provirus usually result in a >10:1 yield of full-length defective to non-defective proviruses. The defective viruses are probably due to mutations that arise in regions of the virus genome essential for function.

Changes that occur in non-essential regions may be tolerated. Examination of variation within individual genes reveals that some regions of the genes are highly variable and others are not. It is clear that the regions of conservation of protein sequences represent functional domains of these proteins. For example, the envelope glycoprotein is, overall, one of the most variable proteins of the virus. However, subregions of this protein include the most conserved in the entire virus and others vary only slightly from strain to strain. Mutational and functional analysis of the envelope glycoprotein shows that the conserved regions encode functions such as CD4 recognition, membrane anchorage, and membrane-to-membrane fusion [56–58].

Viewed from this perspective, natural variation of virus isolates appears to be adventitious. This view accords with the observation that, despite marked sequence variation of HIV isolates, the transmission, pathogenesis, and incubation period of the disease is similar regardless of the infecting strain.

Growth-rate variants may be experimentally selected. Most HIV strains now studied are selected to grow in culture. Viruses that do not grow in culture are difficult to study. It is significant that approximately half of the HIV-1 strains sequenced today are obviously defective in one or both of the negative regulatory genes, *vpu* and *nef*. In addition to mutations that introduce termination codons or that remove initiation codons, it is possible that more subtle damage is present in the regulatory genes of viruses that have been selected to grow in culture. For example, mismatch mutations may be able to produce a full-length protein with reduced activity. It is also conceivable that mutations that accelerate virus growth in culture may occur in the positive as well as negative regulatory pathways. It is likely that the large pool of naturally arising variants that can be found in infected people, particularly during late stages of disease, provides a rich source of variants to be selected by the experimenter.

The rapid rate of variation also raises the possibility that variants of HIV-1 resistant to antiviral drugs may arise in treated patients. The reports of AZT-resistant strains in patients undergoing treatment may reflect selection of such variants [59].

2.13   THE ENVELOPE PROTEIN

The envelope protein of HIV is of interest as it provides a potential target for antiviral drug and vaccine development. Moreover, the envelope glycoprotein has demonstrated to be toxic for CD4+ lymphocytes [60–62].

The envelope protein is made as a single polypeptide chain. It is heavily modified by the addition of complex sugar side-chains via the cellular machinery. The protein is transported to the cell surface and cleaved. The heavily glycosylated amino terminal portion of the protein is located entirely external to the plasma membrane, whereas the more lightly glycosylated carboxy terminus is half in and half out of the membrane and is called the transmembrane protein [2, 3, 62]. The protein is anchored to the membrane by a short lipophilic segment in the centre of the molecule [56].

Dimers and possibly larger aggregates of the *env* protein form via interaction of the exterior portion of the transmembrane protein [63].

The envelope protein specifies two activities, binding to the CD4 cellular surface protein and membrane-to-membrane fusion [56, 58–62, 64] (Fig. 2.11). It is by this means that the virus gains entry to the cell [65, 66]. Cells that express envelope protein will also bind to and fuse with uninfected CD4+ cells. The process of binding and fusion can be reiterated, leading to the formation of giant multinucleated syncytia [60–62] (Figs 2.12(a,b)).

The cytotoxic effect of HIV-1 is dependent on the surface concentration of CD4 as well as on the surface concentration of envelope glycoprotein. Only a low concentration of surface CD4 is needed for infection. However, cells that contain only a small amount of CD4 in the surface are not killed by HIV infection, even when large amounts of the virus are made by such cells [33, 67, 68]. An equation that describes killing of a single cell by HIV-1 is:

$$[\text{virion-associated envelope protein}] \times [\text{CD4}] \times [\text{cell fusion factor}]$$
$$= \text{single cell death}$$

where the term "virion-associated envelope protein" represents the concentration of budding virus that contains a functional envelope glycoprotein protein, the term "CD4" represents the surface concentration of a functional CD4 molecule, and "cell fusion factor" represents the concentration of a cellular factor required for efficient fusion. The latter factor is included in the equation because the effect of the envelope fusion reaction is not solely determined by the surface concentration of CD4. It depends on a property of cells that varies from species to species

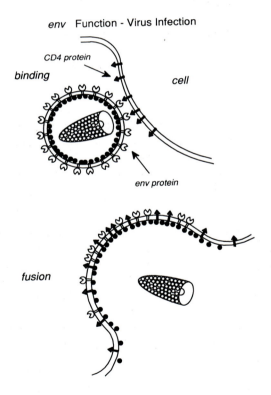

Fig. 2.11 A schematic diagram of the binding and fusion reaction of HIV-1 particle with CD4+ cell.

(a)

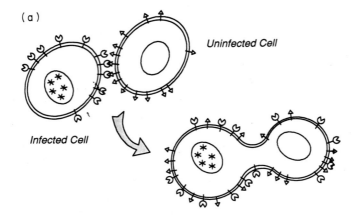

Uninfected Cell

Infected Cell

(b)

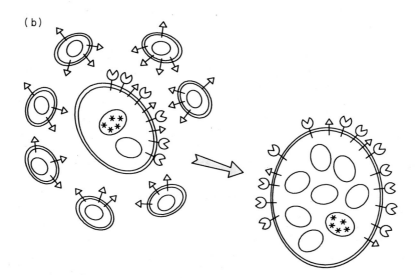

Fig. 2.12 A schematic diagram illustrating (a) the role of the HIV-1 *env* protein in fusion of CD4 cells, and (b) the formation of giant multi-nucleated cells, syncytia.

and even among T lymphoid cell lines of human origin.

Envelope-mediated giant-cell formation also accounts for some cell deaths. The surface concentration of the envelope protein in or on the infected cell and the concentration of CD4 on the uninfected fusion partners determine the ultimate size of syncytia as well as the rate of syncytium formation. Under some conditions, syncytia may include up to 500 nuclei. By this means, a single infected cell, under appropriate conditions, can eliminate several hundred uninfected cells. Death of uninfected cells by syncytium formation may account for the disappearance of a large number of CD4+ T cells in HIV-1 infected patients under conditions in which only one in 10 000 of the CD4 cells express viral antigen. This mechanism may be summarized by the equation

$$[1 \times 10^{-4} \text{ cells expressing viral antigen}]$$
$$\times [100–500 \text{ uninfected CD4+ T cells}] = 1\text{–}5\% \text{ cell death}$$

Large CD4+ virus-infected syncytia have been found in abundance in rhesus macaque monkeys infected with simian immunodeficiency virus (SIV), a virus that is a close relative of HIV-1 [69]. Syncytia are observed in lymph nodes, liver, thymus, spleen, and brain of the infected animals. CD4+ HIV-1 syncytia have also been found on autopsy in the spleens of some HIV-infected people [70]. Abundant syncytia are frequently found in the brain on autopsy of patients that have serious neurological complications of HIV-1 infection [71, 72]. Abundant CD4+ syncytia are not expected to be found in routine autopsies of AIDS patients. Late in disease the number of CD4+ lymphocytes is extremely low [73]. However, the similarity of pathogenesis of SIV and HIV infection indicates that syncytia formation is a significant pathogenic process in humans as well as in monkeys.

The regions of the envelope glycoprotein that specify specific functions have been identified by analysis of the functional consequences of mutations introduced in known positions in the sequences that specify the envelope glycoprotein [56, 58] (Fig. 2.13). The amino-acid sequences that comprise the CD4 binding site are located in three contiguous regions of conserved amino-acid sequence near the carboxy terminus of the exterior glycoprotein. These three regions are postulated to fold into a pocket that serves as a binding site for CD4 (Fig. 2.14). The region that specifies membrane-to-membrane fusion is a short hydrophobic amino-acid sequence near the amino terminus of the transmembrane protein. The short lipophilic sequence near the centre of the transmembrane protein anchors the entire envelope protein to the cell membrane. Two extensive regions near the amino terminus of the two proteins form the interface over which non-covalent attachment of the two subunits occurs.

It is possible to construct a dynamic model for the binding and fusion reactions from this information (Fig. 2.15). Juxtaposition of the two membranes is postulated to occur by high-affinity association between the exterior glycoprotein of one membrane of the CD4 molecule embedded in the second membrane. A binding-induced conformation change is then postulated to occur such that the hydrophobic amino terminus of the transmembrane protein is inserted into the apposed membrane. It is likely that the exterior envelope glycoprotein is displaced at this time. Disruption of the surface of the juxtaposed membranes by the transmembrane protein is postulated to initiate the fusion reaction.

2.14   EVASION OF THE IMMUNE RESPONSE

The structure of the envelope protein and the life-cycle of HIV helps us to understand how the virus evades the immune response. One of the earliest paradoxes regarding HIV infection was that the disease was observed to progress despite an immune response to viral antigens. Progressive disease was particularly puzzling because a high antibody titre to conserved regions on the envelope glycoprotein was reported in early experiments [74, 75]. This paradox was underscored when it was found that most human sera have a very poor ratio of virus-neutralizing activity as compared with the concentration of antibodies that bind the envelope glycoprotein [76, 77]. For example, human sera do not completely inhibit the envelope-mediated syncytium formation reaction [61, 62]. Most sera of HIV-1 infected people have no effect on this reaction, whereas the sera from others only slow the kinetics of syncytium formation. These observations indicate that the immunodominant epitopes of the envelope protein are either not *important* for function or not *accessible* to antibodies when part of a functional envelope protein.

The immunodominant epitopes of HIV-1 have been located [78–81]. They include the carboxy terminus of the exterior glycoprotein, the amino terminal third of the transmembrane protein, and the short-region-located amino terminal of the CD4-binding region of the exterior glycoprotein. Neither the CD4 binding region nor the fusion domain is immunodominant.

The carboxy terminus of the exterior glycoprotein is the site of proteolytic cleavage by a cellular enzyme [2, 62, 82]. For this reason it is very likely to be exposed to the surface. The sequence of the cleavage site is well conserved among HIV-1 isolates [82]. However, antibodies to this region do not inhibit envelope function, whether such antibodies are derived from patient antisera or have been raised to synthetic peptides

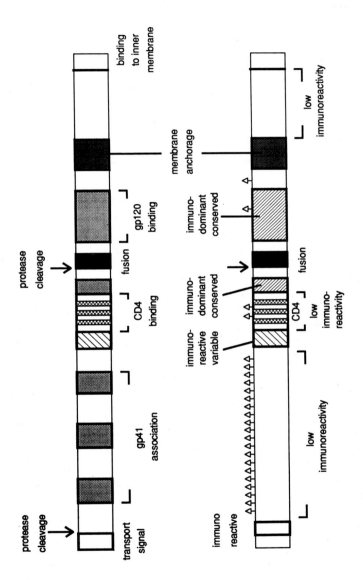

Fig. 2.13 A schematic representation of functional and antigenic regions of the HIV-1 *env* protein.

corresponding to the predicted amino-acid sequence of the region.

The amino terminal third of the transmembrane protein is located at the interface of the exterior and transmembrane envelope proteins. Although the sequence is highly conserved among HIV-1 isolates [83], it is unlikely to be exposed to the surface in the assembled envelope complex. The region will be exposed once the exterior glycoprotein is shed. However, in the assembled functional protein this sequence should be sequestered.

The third immunodominant region is hypervariable in sequence [80].

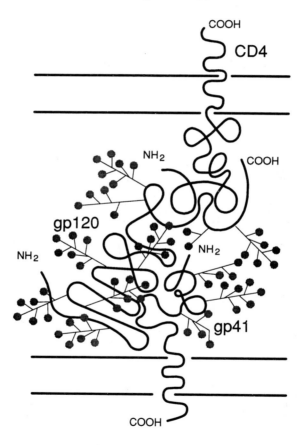

Fig. 2.14 A schematic model of gp120–gp41 CD4 interaction. CD4 is shown embedded in the cell membrane. The HIV-1 *env* protein is shown embedded in the viral membrane. The gp120 protein is shown as a bridge binding to gp41 and to CD4. The sugar side-chains of gp120–gp41 are illustrated.

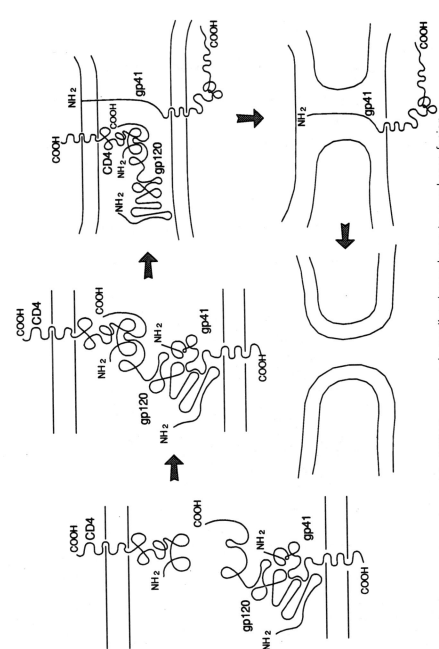

Fig. 2.15 A dynamic model of HIV-1 *env* protein-mediated membrane-to-membrane fusion.

Mutants in this region — located just amino-terminal to the CD4 binding site — are reported to permit resistance to antibodies raised to peptides that correspond in sequence to a particular strain of HIV-1 [84].

The absence of high-titre antibodies to the important functional domains, the CD4 binding region and the fusion region, is a possible consequence of their being sequestered by tertiary folding of the envelope glycoprotein.

Patient antisera do not recognize extensive regions of amino-acid sequence of the exterior glycoprotein. These sequences are heavily covered with complex sugars. The density of sugar residues is predicted to be so great that a contiguous "sugar dome" is expected to be formed over the surface of the protein. The complex sugars are added to the envelope protein by cellular enzyme systems, and for that reason are not antigenic.

In summary, it appears that the envelope protein is constructed to conceal the essential functional domains, either by complex sugar addition or by tertiary conformation.

The ability of the virus to lie dormant as a provirus without expressing viral RNA or protein is another mechanism of evasion of the immune response. In this state, the viral genetic information is invisible to the immune system. Additionally, it is reported that in macrophages HIV-1 virus particles bud to the interior vesicles and are not present on the surface of the cell [85]. In such a case, the infected cell cannot be recognized by the immune system.

These considerations do not mean that it will be impossible to create a vaccine to prevent HIV-1 infection. However, these features of the virus do help to explain the failure of current vaccine attempts, and indicate that effective vaccines must produce antibody responses different from those characteristic of natural infections. One path toward effective vaccines is indicated by the success of blocking HIV infections by reagents that inhibit the envelope glycoprotein–CD4 interaction. Soluble forms of the CD4 surface molecule and monoclonal antibodies that bind to certain epitopes of CD4 completely prevent HIV-1 infection by inhibiting binding of the envelope protein to CD4 [53, 64, 86–90]. The sequences that specify the binding are conserved among HIV-1 strains [56, 58]. Antibody responses in humans that produce similar reactivities should prevent HIV-1 infections. However, such antibody responses may interfere with normal immune function, and must be explored with care.

2.15 SUMMARY

Some of the major features of the acquired immune deficiency syndrome may be understood in terms of the characteristics of the virus. Life-long infection is a consequence of the life-cycle of retroviruses, the formation of stably integrated viral genetic information into host-cell DNA. Silent infection, controlled replication, and prolific replication may be understood in terms of the interactions of the positive and negative regulatory genes that control virus growth. Selective infectivity and selective cytotoxicity of HIV-1 are primarily the consequences of the properties of the envelope glycoprotein and its interactions with the surface CD4 molecule. Concealment of the virus by regulated growth, by budding to the interior surfaces of macrophages, as well as concealment by a sugar coating, may help to explain the failure to protect chimpanzees from infection by candidate vaccines.

Rapid medical prophylaxis is required in populations that currently experience a high incidence of HIV-1 infection. Chemoprevention, the use of chemicals to prevent establishment of viral infection, in addition to vaccination should be investigated as a means to control the AIDS epidemic.

REFERENCES

1. Jacks, T., Power, M.D., Masierz, F.R., Luciw, P.A., Bar, P.J. and Varmus, H.E. (1987). *Nature, Lond.* **331**, 280–283.
2. Robey, W.G., Safai, B., Oroszlan, S. *et al.* (1985). *Science* **228**, 593–595.
3. Allan, J.A., Coligan, J.E., Lee, T.H. *et al.* (1985). *Science* **230**, 810–815.
4. Sodroski, J.G., Goh, W.C., Rosen, C., Dayton, A., Terwilliger, E. and Haseltine, W.A. (1986). *Nature, Lond.* **321**, 412–417.
5. Rabson, A.B. (1990). In *AIDS: Pathogenesis and Treatment* (J.A. Levy, ed.). Marcel Dekker, New York (in press).
6. Ho, D.D., Pomerantz, R.J. and Kaplan, J.C. (1987). *New Engl. J. Med.* **317**, 278.
7. Sodroski, J.G., Rosen, C.A. and Haseltine, W.A. (1984). *Science* **225**, 381.
8. Corden, J., Wasylk, B., Buschwalder, A., Sassone-Corsi, P., Kedinger, C. and Chambon, P. *Science* **209**, 1406–1414.
9. Garcia, J.A., Wa, F.K., Mitsuyasu, R. and Gaynor, R.B. (1980). *EMBO J.* **6**, 3761–3770.
10. Jones, K., Kadonaga, J., Luciw, P. and Tijian, R. (1986). *Science* **232**, 755–759.
11. Nabel, G. and Baltimore, D. (1987). *Nature, Lond.* **326**, 711–713.
12. Rosen, C.A., Sodroski, J.G. and Haseltine, W.A. (1985). *Cell* **4**, 705–716.
13. Shaw, J.P., Uts, P.J., Durand, D.B., Toole, J.J., Emmel, E.A. and

Crabtree, G.R. (1988). *Science* **241**, 202–205.

14. Skevila, M., Josephs, S.F., Dukovich, M., Peffer, N., Wong-Staal, F. and Greene, W.C. (1987). *Science* **238**, 1575–1578.
15. Lu, Y., Stenzel, M., Sodroski, J.G. and Haseltine, W.A. (1989). *J. Virol.* **63**, 4115–4119.
16. Sodroski, J., Rosen, C., Wong-Staal, F. *et al.* (1985). *Science* **227**, 171–173.
17. Dayton, A.I., Sodroski, J.G., Rosen, C.A., Goh, W.C. and Haseltine, W.A. (1986). *Cell* **44**, 941–947.
18. Fisher, A.G., Feinberg, M.B., Josephs, S.F. *et al.* (1986). *Nature, Lond.* **320**, 367–371.
19. Arya, S.K., Guo, C., Joseph, S.F. and Wong-Staal, F. (1985). *Science* **229**, 69–73.
20. Sodroski, J., Patarca, R., Rosen, C. and Haseltine, W.A. (1985). *Science* **229**, 74–77.
21. Hauber, J., Perkins, A., Heimer, E. and Cullen, B. (1987). *Proc. Natl Acad. Sci. USA* **84**, 6364–6368.
22. Ruben, S., Perkins, A., Purcell, R., Joung, K. and Rosen, C.R. (1989). *J. Virol.* **63**, 1–8.
23. Rosen, C.A., Sodroski, J.G. and Haseltine, W.A. (1985). *Cell* **41**, 813–823.
24. Peterlin, B.M., Luciw, P.A., Barr, P.J. and Walker, M.D. (1986). *Proc. Natl Acad. Sci. USA* **83**, 9734–9738.
25. Hauber, J. and Cullen, B. (1988). *J. Virol.* **62**, 673.
26. Muesing, M.A., Smith, D.H. and Capon, D.J. (1987). *Cell* **48**, 691.
27. Patarca, R. and Haseltine, W.E. (1987). *AIDS Res. Hum. Retroviruses* **3**, 1.
28. Feng, S. and Holland, E.C. (1988). *Nature, Lond.* **334**, 165.
29. Rosen, C.A., Sodroski, J.G., Goli, W.L., Dayton, A.L., Lipke, J. and Haseltine, W.A. (1986). *Nature, Lond.* **319**, 555–559.
30. Wright, C.M., Felber, B.K., Paskalis, H. and Pavlakis, G.N. (1986). *Science* **234**, 988.
31. Cullen, B. (1986) *Cell* **46**, 973.
32. Sodroski, J.G., Goli, W.C., Rosen, C., Dayton, A., Terwilliger, E. and Haseltine, W.A. (1986). *Nature, Lond.* **321**, 412–417.
33. Feinberg, M.B., Jarret, R.F., Aldovini, A., Gallo, R.C. and Wong-Staal, F. (1986). *Cell* **46**, 807–817.
34. Terwilliger, E.F., Sodroski, J.G., Haseltine, W.A. and Rosen, C.A. (1988). *J. Virol.* **62**, 655–658.
35. Rosen, C.A., Terwilliger, E., Dayton, A., Sodroski, J.G. and Haseltine, W.A. (1988). *Proc. Natl Acad. Sci. USA* **85**, 2071–2075.
36. Malin, M.H., Hauber, J., Fenrick, R. and Cullen, B.R. (1988). *Nature, Lond.* **335**, 181–183.
37. Emerman, M., Vazeux, R. and Peden, K. (1989). *Cell* **67**, 1155–1165.
38. Knight, D.M., Floerfelt, F.A. and Ghrayeb, J. (1987). *Science* **236**, 837–840.
39. Allan, J.S., Coligan, J.F., Barin, F. *et al.* (1985). *Science* **228**, 1091–1094.
40. Fischer, A.G., Ratner, L., Mitsuya, H. *et al.* (1986). *Science* **233**, 655–658.
41. Terwilliger, E., Sodroski, J.G., Rosen, C.A. and Haseltine, W.A. (1986). *J. Virol.* **60**, 754–760.
42. Luciw, P.A., Cheng-Mayer, C. and Levy, J.A. (1987). *Proc. Natl Acad. Sci. USA* **84**, 1434–1438.
43. Muesing, M.A., Smith, D.H., Cabradilla, C.D., Benton, C.V., Lasky, L.A. and Capon, D.J. (1985). *Nature, Lond.* **313**, 480–488.

44. Fisher, A.G., Ratner, L., Matsuya, H. *et al.* (1987). *Science* **237**, 888.
45. Guy, B., Kieny, M.P., Riviere, Y. *et al.* (1987). *Nature, Lond.* **330**, 266–269.
46. Lee, T.H., Coligan, J.E., Allan, J.S., McLane, M.F., Groopman, J.E. and Essex, M. (1986). *Science* **231**, 1546–1549.
47. Sodroski, J., Goli, W.C., Rosen, C. *et al.* (1988). *Science* **231**, 159–163.
48. Strebel, K., Daugherty, D., Clouse, K., Cohen, D., Folks, T. and Martin, M.A. (1987). *Nature, Lond.* **328**, 728.
49. Strebel, K., Klimkait, T. and Martin, M.A. (1988). *Science* **241**, 1221–1223.
50. Cohen, E.A., Terwilliger, E.F., Sodroski, J.G. and Haseltine, W.A. (1988). *Nature, Lond.* **334**, 532–534.
51. Terwilliger, E.F., Cohen, E.A., Lu, Y., Sodroski, J.G. and Haseltine, W.A. (1989). *Proc. Natl Acad. Sci. USA* **86**, 5163–5167.
52. Barre-Sinoussi, F., Chermann, J.C., Rey, F. *et al.* (1983). *Science* **220**, 868–871.
53. Klatzmann, D., Champagne, E., Chamaret, S. *et al.* (1984). *Nature, Lond.* **312**, 767–768.
54. Popovic, M., Sarngadharan, M.G., Read, E. and Gallo, R.C. (1984). *Science* **224**, 497–500.
55. Harper, M.E., Marsell, L.M., Gallo, R.C. and Wong-Staal, F. (1986). *Proc. Natl Acad. Sci. USA* **83**, 772–776.
56. Kowalski, M., Potz, J., Basiripour, L. *et al.* (1987). *Science* **237**, 1351–1355.
57. Jameson, B.A., Rao, P.E., Kahn, L.I. *et al.* (1988). *Science* **240**, 1335–1339.
58. Lasky, L., Nakamura, G., Smith, D. *et al.* (1987). *Cell* **50**, 975–985.
59. Larder, B.A., Darby, G. and Richman, D.D. (1989). *Science* **243**, 1731–1734.
60. Lifson, J., Feinberg, M., Reyes, G. *et al.* (1986). *Nature, Lond.* **323**, 725–728.
61. Lifson, J., Reyes, G., McGrath, M., Stein, B. and Engleman, E. (1986). *Science* **232**, 1123–1127.
62. Sodroski, J., Goli, W.C., Rosen, C., Campbell, K. and Haseltine, W.A. (1986). *Nature, Lond.* **322**, 470–474.
63. Pinter, A., Honnen, W.J., Tilley, S.A. *et al.* (1989). *J. Virol.* **63**, 2674–2679.
64. McDougal, J., Kennedy, M., Sligh, J., Cort, S., Mawle, A. and Nicholson, J. (1986). *Science* **231**, 382–385.
65. Stein, B., Gowda, S., Lifson, J., Penhallow, R., Bensch, K. and Engelman, E. (1987). *Cell* **49**, 659–668.
66. Bedinger, P., Moriarty, A., Von Borstel, R.C., Donovan, N.J., Steimer, K.S. and Littman, D.R. (1988). *Nature, Lond.* **334**, 162–165.
67. Gartner, S., Markovits, P., Markovitz, D.M., Kaplan, M.H., Gallo, R.C. and Popovic, M. (1986). *Science* **233**, 215–219.
68. DeRossi, A., Franchini, G., Aldovini, A., Del Mistro, A., Chieco-Bianchi, L., Gallo, R. and Wong-Staal, F. (1986). *Proc. Natl Acad. Sci. USA* **83**, 4297–4301.
69. Benveniste, R., Morton, W., Clark, E. *et al.* (1988). *J. Virol.* **62**, 2091–2101.
70. Byrnes, R.K., Chan, W.C., Spira, T.J., Ewing, E.P. and Chandler, F.W. (1983). *J. Am. Med. Assoc.* **250**, 1313–1317.
71. Price, R., Brew, B., Sidtis, J., Rosenblum, M., Scheck, A. and Cleary, P. (1988). *Science* **239**, 586–592.
72. Nielson, S.L., Petito, C.K., Urmacher, D.C. and Posner, J.B. (1984). *Am. J. Clin. Pathol.* **82**, 678.
73. Ewing, E.P., Chandler, F.W., Spira, T.J., Byrnes, R.K. and Chan, W.C.

(1985). *Arch. Pathol. Lab. Med.* **109**, 977–981.
74. Barin, F., McLane, M.F., Allan, J.S., Lee, T.H., Groopman, J. and Essex, M. (1985). *Science* **228**, 1094–1096.
75. Sarngadharan, M., Popovic, M., Bruch, L., Schupbach, J. and Gallo, R.C. (1984). *Science* **224**, 506–508.
76. Weiss, R., Clapham, P., Cheingsong-Popov, R. *et al.* (1985). *Nature, Lond.* **316**, 69–72.
77. Robert-Guroff, M., Brown, M. and Gallo, R.C. (1985). *Nature, Lond.* **316**, 72–74.
78. Matthews, T., Langlois, A., Robey, W. *et al.* (1986). *Proc. Natl Acad. Sci. USA* **83**, 9709–9713.
79. Gann, J., Nelson, J. and Oldstone, M. (1987). *J. Virol.* **61**, 2639–2641.
80. Palker, T., Matthews, T., Clark, M. *et al.* (1987). *Proc. Natl Acad. Sci. USA* **84**, 2479–2483.
81. Wang, J., Steel, S., Wisniewolski, R. and Wang, C. (1986). *Proc. Natl Acad. Sci. USA* **83**, 6159–6163.
82. McCune, J., Rabin, L. Feinberg, M. *et al.* (1988). *Cell* **53**, 55–67.
83. Gallagher, W.R. (1987). *Cell* **50**, 327.
84. Looney, D., Fisher, A., Putney, S. *et al.* (1988). *Science* **241**, 357–359.
85. Orenstein, J., Meltzer, M., Phipps, T. and Gendelman, H. (1988). *J. Virol.* **62**, 2578–2586.
86. Deen, K.C., McDougal, J.S., Inacker, R. *et al.* (1988). *Nature, Lond.* **331**, 82–84.
87. Hussey, R., Richardson, N., Kowalski, M. *et al.* (1988). *Nature, Lond.* **331**, 76–79.
88. Traunecker, A., Luke, W. and Karjalainen, K. (1988). *Nature, Lond.* **331**, 84–86.
89. Smith, D., Byrn, R., Marsters, S., Gregory, T., Groopman, J. and Capon, D. (1987). *Science* **238**, 1704–1707.
90. Sattentau, Q., Dalgleish, A., Weiss, R. and Beverly, P. (1986). *Science* **234**, 1120–1123.

3 | Molecular Interactions Between CD4 and the HIV Envelope Glycoproteins

QUENTIN J. SATTENTAU

Academic Department of Genito-Urinary Medicine, University College and Middlesex School of Medicine, Cleveland Street, London W1, UK

3.1 CD4 IS THE HIV CELLULAR RECEPTOR

Since the isolation of the causative agent of AIDS, the human immunodeficiency virus (HIV) in 1983, an enormous body of work has accumulated describing all aspects of the immunology and virology of HIV infection. One of the areas which has received most attention is the interaction of HIV with its cellular receptor, the CD4 antigen [1]. In initial studies, several lines of evidence implicated CD4 as the HIV receptor: (a) human peripheral blood lymphocytes bearing CD4 but not CD8 are permissive for infection [2]; (b) monoclonal antibodies (mAbs) to CD4 but not to other cell surface antigens block HIV infection and cell fusion [3, 4]; (c) the HIV major envelope glycoprotein gp120 can be coprecipitated with CD4 from infected cells [5], and recombinant forms of gp120 bind to CD4 with high affinity [6]; and (d) transfection of CD4 cDNA into CD4-human cell lines renders them susceptible to HIV infection [7]. Subsequent studies have confirmed and extended these findings, and more recently considerable effort has been put into the genetic manipulation of the CD4 gene to define precisely those regions interactive with gp120 and MHC class II antigens. Several laboratories are currently focusing on events subsequent to HIV receptor binding, particularly with regard to virus–cell fusion, and mechanisms of HIV pathogenesis and tissue tropism are receiving considerable attention.

A number of recent studies have also demonstrated that CD4 may have an important role in signal transduction, based on the association with the p56lck tyrosine kinase. Aspects of normal CD4 function such as this will not be addressed here, but are dealt with in detail in several recent and thorough reviews [8–10].

AIDS AND THE NEW VIRUSES
ISBN 0-12-200740-9

3.2   MAPPING OF FUNCTIONAL SITES ON CD4

The CD4 molecule consists of an extracellular segment containing four immunoglobulin-like domains followed by a membrane spanning region and a cytoplasmic tail. On this basis CD4 has been included as a member of the immunoglobulin superfamily [11–13]. Within the last few years a number of laboratories have attempted to define those regions of CD4 which bind to gp120. Initial studies using monoclonal antibodies (mAbs) to define epitopes which are important in HIV-1, HIV-2 and SIV infectivity and cell fusion demonstrated that those mAbs reactive with the N-terminal regions of CD4, of which Leu3a, OKT4A and MT151 are prototypes, were the most potent inhibitors of the virus–receptor interaction, whereas other mAbs such as OKT4, which bind to a more C-terminal region, were inactive in these assays [14, 15]. Interestingly, a number of mAbs which clustered with Leu3a on the basis of cross-competition studies and were potent inhibitors of HIV binding also recognised highly conserved epitopes of non-human primate CD4 molecules, suggesting an important functional significance for this region [16]. Genetic manipulation of the CD4 gene has since allowed detailed mutational analyses of regions and single amino acids important in gp120 binding. Truncation of the CD4 cDNA at the transmembrane region has resulted in the production of a secreted, soluble form of the molecule (sCD4) which retains full binding to gp120, and thus has potential therapeutic value (for reviews see Doyle et al. in [9], and Chapter 4 in this book). Similarly, termination of CD4 at the end of the second domain has resulted in the expression of polypeptides consisting of the first 179 amino acids which also retain maximal binding [17–19], and in a thorough study [19] Arthos and colleagues have unequivocally demonstrated that the first 106 amino acids approximating to the N-terminal disulphide linked domain of CD4 has affinity for gp120 equivalent to that of sCD4. At present this appears to be the smallest subunit which still retains high affinity binding, since synthetic peptides prepared from sections of V1 have little or no reactivity for gp120 (unpublished results). More detailed mapping analyses of the interactive sites have taken two forms: peptide mapping and site-specific mutation of the CD4 gene. Jameson and colleagues [20] proposed a model for the N-terminal domain of CD4 based on the binding of a panel of HIV-blocking CD4 mAbs to peptides, in which the HIV binding site was proposed to be a loop projecting from the surface of the molecule spanning residues 37–53. Other studies based on inhibition of HIV infection and cell fusion by benzylated peptides defined a second region within domain 1, residues 76–94 [21, 22]. These peptide derivatives probably define the CDR3 region of V1 as functional in HIV entry rather than virus binding, although the significance of these findings is unclear since when purified to homogeneity, no activity remained. Several mutational analyses have more precisely defined critical regions and residues within the first domain. Various strategies have been adopted in these studies: saturation mutagenesis followed by negative and positive antibody selection [23]; substitution of stretches of human CD4 sequence onto a mouse background [24, 25] or site-directed substitution of individual or clusters of residues against a murine template [19, 26]; and linker insertion [27]. The core sequence interacting with gp120 as defined by these studies spans residues 41–55. The sequence identity of the first domain of CD4 with that of immunoglobulin variable light chain domains has allowed prediction of the tertiary structure, and several groups have proposed models based on the folding of the Bence–Jones light chain homodimer, REI [19, 20, 24, 28, 29]. The conclusions from these studies are in general agreement that the binding site for gp120 corresponds to a region analagous to the CDR-2 loop and supporting B-strands of a Vk light chain domain (Fig. 3.1). There is speculation, based on the inability to detect an antibody response in HIV seropositive individuals or gp120 immunized animals against the gp120 binding site, that this region may be a narrow cleft inaccessible to immunoglobulin molecules, as previously proposed for rhinoviruses [30]. This idea would suggest that the active site on CD4 might be a loop projecting away from the main bulk of the molecule, as proposed by Jameson *et al.* [20], although another study does not support a projecting loop, but perhaps a face [29]. Clearly the elucidation of structural details such as this will have to wait until the atomic structure is determined by X-ray crystallography.

Two groups have recently attempted to compare the regions of CD4 important for gp120 binding with those critical for interaction with MHC class II antigens. Overexpression of CD4 molecules on transfected cells can result in rosette formation with MHC class II-expressing cell lines such as B-lymphoblastoid lines [31]. This assay has been exploited to determine those amino-acid substitutions in CD4 which eliminate rosetting [32–34]. Both studies show that binding of these two ligands to CD4 is separable by distinct mutations: gp120 binding is only eliminated by mutations in the CDR-2 loop and supporting strands of the first domain, whereas MHC class II binding is affected by a number of mutations in the first, second and third domains. This implies that the construction of small CD4-binding molecules that inhibit gp120 binding, but do not interfere with MHC class II interactions, is a possibility.

(a)

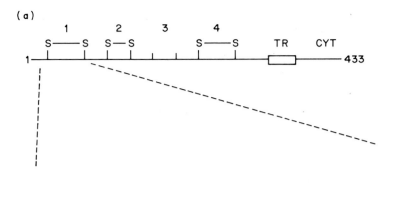

(b)

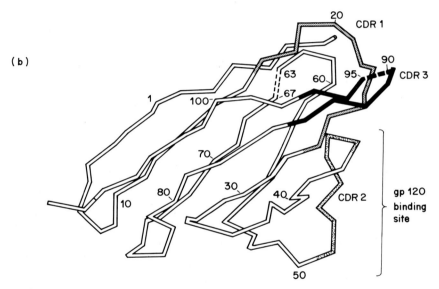

Fig. 3.1   (a) The proposed structure of CD4. The extracellular region (amino acids 1–370) contains the immunoglobulin-like domains which are numbered 1–4. The transmembrane segment is represented by TR (371–392) and the cytoplasmic tail is CYT (393–433). gp120 binds within the first domain. (b) Binding region of HIV gp120 on the first domain of CD4. The alpha carbon backbone of CD4 domain 1 indicating the loops corresponding to complementarity determining regions (CDRs) of an Ig Vk domain, and the proposed gp120 binding site spanning residues 42–55 of CDR-2.

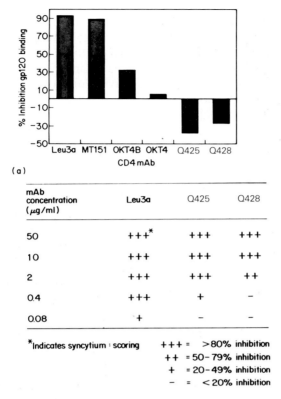

(a)

mAb concentration (μg/ml)	Leu3a	Q425	Q428
50	+++*	+++	+++
10	+++	+++	+++
2	+++	+++	++
0.4	+++	+	-
0.08	+	-	-

*Indicates syncytium ÷ scoring   +++ = >80% inhibition
                                         ++ = 50-79% inhibition
                                          + = 20-49% inhibition
(b)   - = <20% inhibition

Fig. 3.2 (a) Inhibition of gp120 binding by CD4 mAbs. Recombinant gp120 (2 μg/ml) was reacted with the CD4+ T cell line SUPT1 in the presence or absence of 10 μg/ml of CD4 mAb, then detected with ^{125}I-labelled anti-gp120 mAb. Binding of gp120 was taken as 100% without inhibitory mAbs present, and 0% in the absence of gp120. Leu3a and MT151, which bind within the first domain and first and second domains, respectively, block strongly; OKT4B, which binds only in the second domain, blocks weakly; OKT4, Q425 and Q428, which bind outside the first two domains, do not inhibit gp120 binding. (b) Inhibition of HIV-induced syncytium formation by CD4 mAbs Q425 and Q428. Inhibition by Q425 is about five-fold, and Q428 about 25-fold, less than Leu3a.

3.3   HIV ENTRY INTO CD4+ CELLS

There are two recognized mechanisms of enveloped virus entry into receptor-bearing cells: pH-dependent (as for orthomyxo-, rhabdo- and togaviruses) fusion of virus particles with the membrane of endocytic vesicles, or pH-independent fusion directly with the plasma membrane (paramyxoviruses, see review [35]). An initial study reported that receptor-mediated endocytosis might play a significant role in HIV entry [7], but subsequent studies have not supported this as a major mechanism of virus internalization. In two reports in which inhibitors of the endocytic pathway were included in HIV infectivity or syncytium assays, no significant reduction in virus infection or fusion was observed [36, 37]. Bedinger and colleagues [38] have expressed truncated or chimaeric forms of CD4 in a CD4− human cell line. These molecules were not internalized by phorbol ester (a potent inducer of endocytosis of native CD4) but were still effective receptors for HIV infection. Similar results have been obtained by Maddon et al. using deletion or serine substitution in the cytoplasmic domain of CD4, and additional data showed that native CD4 does not appear to enter the cell with HIV [39]. It is unclear whether CD4 is necessary simply for virus attachment, or whether it plays a more complex role and is involved in HIV entry. A chimaeric molecule consisting of the first two domains of CD4 linked to the hinge, transmembrane and cytoplasmic segments of CD8 conferred susceptibility to a CD4− T cell line [38], demonstrating that the third and fourth domains of CD4 are unnecessary for HIV infection and that CD8 can substitute for CD4 in this region. That the gp120 binding domain of CD4 is sufficient to allow infection of permissive cells has yet to be demonstrated, however. The possibility that CD4 may be necessary for events leading to infection subsequent to virus binding is implied by three sets of data: (1) CD4 mAbs prepared in our laboratory which bind outside the gp120 reactive region and hence do not interfere with gp120 binding are potently able to inhibit HIV infectivity and cell fusion (Fig. 2 and Table 1 in [40]). At present the mechanism of such an effect is unclear, but may relate to alteration of CD4 conformation resulting in a non-permissive form; (2) a very recent study by Camerini and Seed [41] demonstrates that CD4 cloned from chimpanzee lymphocytes and expressed in HeLa cells is unable to mediate syncytium formation with HIV env-expressing cells. Substitution of amino acids in human CD4 with the equivalent residues in the chimp sequence defined residue 87 in the CDR3 region of V1 as critical for syncytium formation, but had no effect on gp120 binding. Interestingly the syncytium incompetent clone of CD4 mediated infection of HeLa cells with HIV, suggesting that there may be either qualitative or substantial quantitative differences between cell–cell fusion and virus–cell fusion; (3) the binding of soluble, recombinant CD4 to HIV-infected cells results in increased shedding of gp120 into the supernatant, which may reflect a CD4-triggered mechanism for the exposure of masked fusogenic sites on gp41 (J. Moore, J. McKeating and

R. A. Weiss, Chester-Beatty Laboratories, London, unpublished results).

The finding that both HIV and VSV(HIV) pseudotypes are unable to infect mouse cells expressing human CD4 [7] has been taken as evidence to suggest that either there is a second factor required in addition to CD4 to achieve infection, or that mouse cells and cells of other non-primate mammals (P. Clapham and R.A. Weiss, unpublished results) contain an element suppressive to HIV entry. In accord with this latter hypothesis is the finding that somatic cell hybrids between human and mouse cells which span the full complement of human chromosomes and express human CD4 are not permissive for HIV infection [42]. Other studies concerned with the ability of SIV to infect only a restricted number of CD4+ human cell lines demonstrate that CD4 expression is not always sufficient to allow infection and cell fusion, and conclude that additional elements are required [43, 44]. A number of laboratories are actively seeking such factors by a variety of strategies. Recent reports describing the potential involvement of a cell surface protease in HIV syncytium formation may indeed be such a molecule, facilitating HIV infection by proteolytic cleavage of a critical region of gp120 [45, 46].

3.4   THE gp120–CD4 INTERACTION IN THE PATHOGENESIS OF HIV INFECTION

Although the proposed MHC class II interactive site on CD4 is different from the gp120 binding site, they overlap and hence gp120 bound to cellular CD4 would be expected to interfere with MHC class II-dependent T cell activation. This is clearly the case, as has been shown by *in vitro* studies [47, 48], although evidence to support this *in vivo*, such as the detection of gp120 bound to CD4+ lymphocytes in HIV-infected individuals, is lacking. One factor which would determine whether these mechanisms occur *in vivo* is whether there is sufficient soluble gp120 shed from virus particles and HIV-infected cells to coat CD4+ T lymphocytes. This seems unlikely to take place in the periphery, but may occur in tissues where there is a higher density of HIV-infected cells, such as lymph nodes. A very recent study addresses the issue of low levels of soluble gp120 inhibiting T cell activation [49], and demonstrates that gp120 bound to CD4+ cells can react synergistically with serum gp120 antibodies forming an immunosuppressive immune complex. This scenario may explain the defect observed in the response of CD4+ lymphocytes from HIV-infected patients [50] to soluble antigens. A consequence of the coating of CD4+ cells with gp120–anti-gp120 may be to affect thymic development of immature double-positive T cells. Bound gp120 may mask CD4 in much the same way as has been shown for CD4 antibodies, preventing the positive selection of CD4+ MHC class II-restricted T cells [51].

Alternative mechanisms of gp120-mediated immunopathogenesis have been proposed that also rely less on the quantity of gp120 adsorbed to the CD4+ cell. These are based on gp120 bound to CD4 as a target for antibody-dependent cell-mediated cytotoxicity (ADCC) [52], or peptides of gp120 presented by MHC class II on CD4+ T cells to CD4+ cytotoxic T cell lines [53, 54]. An argument against these mechanisms is that if a large number of CD4+ T cells were being destroyed as a result of binding gp120, then other gp120 binding cells would also be destroyed, such as monocyte/macrophages and gp120-specific B cells, for which there is little evidence. One important factor limiting studies of HIV pathogenesis is the availability of relevant animal models. It may be that the severe combined immunodeficiency mouse reconstituted with the human immune system (SCID-Hu mouse) [55] will help greatly in elucidating mechanisms of HIV pathogenicity.

3.5   TROPISM OF HIV FOR CD4 BEARING CELLS

The earliest observation of HIV tissue tropism was the destruction of CD4+ T cells in AIDS patients. Subsequent studies revealed that other cell types bearing CD4 were infected in seropositive individuals, most notably those of the myeloid lineage: monocyte/macrophages [56], microglia [57, 58] and Langerhans cells [59]. All of these cell types can be infected in vitro, as can certain other CD4+ cell lines of different origin, such as EBV-transformed B cell lines [60, 61], colon carcinoma cells and fibroblasts [60]. The addition of HIV to glioma cell lines [62–64] and primary glial cell cultures [65] leads to low-level infection which can be detected by sensitive techniques such as co-cultivation with susceptible CD4+ target cells. Although CD4 has been detected either on the surface or at the mRNA level in glial cell cultures by some groups [65, 66], others have reported failure to detect CD4 expression in any form, and are unable to block HIV infection of these cultures using CD4 mAbs or soluble CD4 [64, 67]. The relevance of these findings to the situation in vivo is, however, unclear since: (1) there is no evidence for HIV antigens or mRNA in neural tissues from infected individuals other than in microglia or perivascular macrophages [57, 58]; and (2) no cytopathic effect has been seen in infected glial cell cultures or in neural tissues other than macrophage-derived cells. Similar arguments may also apply to the reports of HIV infection of colon carcinoma cell lines and fibroblasts [62].

If these tissues do, however, form a non-CD4 expressing HIV reservoir, this may have important implications for any therapies based on interference with the gp120–CD4 interaction.

REFERENCES

1. Sattentau, Q.J. and Weiss, R.A. (1988). The CD4 antigen: physiological ligand and HIV receptor. *Cell* **52**, 631–633.
2. Klatzmann, D., Barre-Sinoussi, F., Nugeyre, M.-T. *et al.* (1984). Selective tropism of lymphadenopathy associated virus (LAV) for helper-inducer T lymphocytes. *Science* **225**, 59–63.
3. Dalgleish, A.G., Beverley, P.C.L., Clapham, P.R., Crawford, D.H., Greaves, M.F. and Weiss, R.A. (1984). The CD4 (T4) antigen is an essential component of the receptor for the AIDS retrovirus. *Nature, Lond.* **312**, 763–767.
4. Klatzmann, D., Champagne, E., Chamaret, S. *et al.* (1984). T-lymphocyte T4 molecule behaves as the receptor for human retrovirus LAV. *Nature, Lond.* **312**, 767–768.
5. McDougal, S., Kennedy, M.S., Sligh, J.M., Cort, S.P., Mawle, A. and Nicholson, J.K. (1986). Binding of HTLV-III/LAV toT4+ T cells by a complex of the 100K viral protein and the T4 molecule. *Science* **231**, 382–385.
6. Lasky, L.A., Nakamura, G., Smith, D.H. *et al.* (1987). Delineation of a region of the immunodeficiency virus type 1 gp120 glycoprotein critical for interaction with the CD4 receptor. *Cell* **50**, 975–985.
7. Maddon, P.J., Dalgleish, A.G., McDougal, J.S., Clapham, P.R., Weiss, R.A. and Axel, R. (1986). The T4 gene encodes the AIDS virus receptor and is expressed in the immune system and the brain. *Cell* **47**, 333–348.
8. Janeway, C.A. Jr. (1989). The role of CD4 in T-cell activation: accessory molecule or co-receptor? *Immunology Today* **10**, 234–238.
9. Function of CD structures on lymphocytes (1989). *Immunol. Rev.* **109** (Ed. G. Moller, Publ. Munksgaard).
10. Rudd, C.E., Anderson, P., Morimoto, C., Streuli, M. and Schlossman, S. (1989). Molecular interactions, T-cell subsets and a role of the CD4/CD8:p56Ick complex in human T-cell activation. *Immunol. Rev.* **111**, 224–266.
11. Clark, S.J., Jeffries, W.A., Barclay, A.N., Gagnon, J. and Williams, A.F. (1987). Peptide and nucleotide sequences of rat CD4 (W3/25) antigen: evidence for derivation from a structure with four immunoglobulin related domains. *Proc. Natl Acad. Sci. USA* **84**, 1649–1653.
12. Maddon, P.J., Molinaux, S.M., Maddon, D.E. *et al.* (1987). Structure and expression of the human and mouse T4 genes. *Proc. Natl Acad. Sci. USA* **84**, 9155–9159.
13. Williams, A.F., Davis, S.J., He, Q. and Barclay, N. (1990). Structural diversity in domains of the immunoglobulin superfamily. *Cold Spring Harbour Symp.* (In press).
14. Sattentau, Q.J., Dalgleish, A.G., Weiss, R.A. and Beverley, P.C.L. (1986). Epitopes of the CD4 antigen and HIV infection. *Science* **234**, 1120–1123.

15. Sattentau, Q.J., Clapham, P.R., Weiss, R.A. *et al.* (1988). The human and simian immunodeficiency viruses HIV-1, HIV-2 and SIV interact with similar epitopes on their cellular receptor, the CD4 molecule. *AIDS* **2**, 101–105.

16. McClure, M.O., Sattentau, Q.J., Beverley, P.C.L. *et al.* (1987). Infection of primate lymphocytes and conservation of the CD4 receptor. *Nature, Lond.* **330**, 487–489.

17. Traunecker, A., Luke, W. and Karjelainers, K. (1988). Soluble CD4 molecules neutralise human immunodeficiency virus type 1. *Nature, Lond.* **331**, 84–86.

18. Berger, E.A., Fuerst, T.R. and Moss, B. (1988). A recombinant polypeptide comprising the amino terminal half of the extracellular region of the CD4 molecule contains an active binding site for human immunodeficiency virus. *Proc. Natl Acad. Sci. USA* **85**, 2357–2361.

19. Arthos, J., Deen, C.K., Chaikin, M.A. *et al.* (1989). Identification of the residues in human CD4 critical for the binding of HIV. *Cell* **57**, 469–481.

20. Jameson, B.A., Rao, P.E., Kong, L.I. *et al.* (1988). Location and chemical synthesis for the binding site for HIV-1 on the CD4 protein. *Science* **240**, 1335–1339.

21. Lifson, J.D., Hwang, K.M., Nara, P.L. *et al.* (1988). Synthetic CD4 peptide derivatives that inhibit HIV infection and cytopathicity. *Science* **241**, 712–716.

22. Nara, P.L., Hwang, K.M., Rausch, D.M., Lifson, J.D. and Eiden, L.E. (1989). CD4 antigen-based antireceptor peptides inhibit infectivity of human immunodeficiency virus *in vitro* at multiple stages of the virus life cycle. *Proc. Natl Acad. Sci. USA* **86**, 7139–7143.

23. Peterson, A. and Seed, B. (1988). Genetic analysis of monoclonal antibody and HIV binding sites on the human lymphocyte antigen CD4. *Cell* **54**, 65–72.

24. Landau, N.R., Wharton, M. and Littman, D.R. (1988). The envelope glycoprotein of the human immunodeficiency virus binds to the immunoglobulin-like domain of CD4. *Nature, Lond.* **334**, 159–162.

25. Estess, P., Salmon, S.L., Winberg, M., Ol, V.T. and Buck, D. (1990). Molecular mapping of immunogenic determinants on human CD4 using chimaeric interspecies molecules and anti CD4 antibodies. In: *Current Research in Protein Chemistry* (Ed. J. Villafranca), Academic Press, New York.

26. Clayton, L.K., Hussey, R.E., Steinbrich, R., Ramachandran, H., Hussain, Y. and Reinherz, E.L. (1988). Substitution of murine for human CD4 residues identifies amino acids critical for HIV-gp120 binding. *Nature, Lond.* **335**, 363–366.

27. Mizukami, T., Fuerst, T.R., Berger, E.A. and Moss, B. (1988). Binding region for human immunodeficiency virus (HIV) and epitopes for HIV blocking monoclonal antibodies of the CD4 molecule defined by site directed mutagenesis. *Proc. Natl Acad. Sci. USA* **85**, 9273–9277.

28. Sattentau, Q.J., Arthos, J., Deen, K. *et al.* (1989). Structural analysis of the human immunodeficiency virus-binding domain of CD4. *J. Exp. Med.* **170**, 198–209.

29. Bates, P.A., McGregor, M.J., Islam, S.A., Sattentau, Q.J. and Sternberg, M.J.E. (1989). A predicted three-dimensional structure for the human

immunodeficiency virus binding domains of CD4 antigen. *Prot. Eng.* **3**, 13–21.

30. Rossman, M.G., Arnold, E., Erickson, J.W. *et al.* (1985). *Nature, Lond.* **317**, 145–152.
31. Doyle, C. and Strominger, J. (1987). Interaction between CD4 and MHC class-II molecules mediates cell adhesion. *Nature, Lond.* **330**, 256–259.
32. Clayton, L.K., Sieh, M., Pious, D.H. and Reinherz, E.L. (1989). Identification of human CD4 residues affecting class II MHC versus HIV-1 gp120 binding. *Nature, Lond.* **339**, 548–551.
33. Lamarre, D., Ashkenazi, A., Fleury, S., Smith, D.H., Sekaly, R-P. and Capon, D.J. (1989). The MHC-binding and gp120-binding functions of CD4 are separable. *Science* **245**: 743–746.
34. Lamarre, D., Capon, D.J., Karp, D.R., Gregory, T., Long, E.O. and Sekaly, R-P. (1989). Class II MHC molecules and the HIV gp120 envelope protein interact with functionally distinct regions of the CD4 molecule. *EMBO J.* **8**, 3271–3277.
35. White, J., Kiellan, M. and Helenius, A. (1983). Membrane fusion proteins of enveloped animal viruses. *Q. Rev. Biophys.* **16**, 151–195.
36. Stein, B.S., Gourda, S.D., Lifson, J.D., Penhallow, R.C., Beusch, K.G. and Engleman, E.G. (1987). pH independent entry into CD4 positive T cells via virus envelope fusion to the plasma membrane. *Cell* **49**, 659–668.
37. McClure, M.O., Marsh, M. and Weiss, R.A. (1988). Human immunodeficiency virus infection of CD4 bearing cells occurs by a pH independent mechanism. *EMBO J.* **7**, 513–516.
38. Bedinger, P., Moriarty, A., von Borstel, R.C.II., Donovan, N.J., Steimer, K.S. and Littman, D.R. (1988). Internalisation of the human immunodeficiency virus does not require the cytoplasmic domain of CD4. *Nature, Lond.* **334**, 162–165.
39. Maddon, P.J., McDougal, J.S., Clapham, P.R. *et al.* (1988). HIV infection does not require endocytosis of its receptor, CD4. *Cell* **54**, 865–874.
40. Healey, D., Dianda, L., McDougal, S.J., Moore, M. *et al.* (1990). HIV infection and fusion of CD4+ cells can be separated from virus binding by CD4 monoclonal antibodies. *J. Exp. Med.* (submitted).
41. Camerini, D. and Seed, B. (1990). A CD4 domain important for HIV-mediated syncytium formation lies outside the virus binding site. *Cell* **60**, 747–754.
42. Tersmette, M., van Dongen, J., Clarham, P. *et al.* (1989). Human immunodeficiency virus infection studied in CD4 expressing human–murine T cell hybrids. *Virology* **168**, 267–273.
43. Hoxie, J.A., Haggarty, B.S., Bonser, S.E., Rackowski, J.L., Shan, H. and Kanki, P. (1988). Biological characterisation of a simian immunodeficiency virus-like retrovirus (HTLV-IV): evidence for CD4 associated molecules required for infection. *J. Virol.* **62**, 2557–2568.
44. Koenig, S., Hirsch, V.M., Olmstead, R.A. *et al.* (1989). Selective infection of human CD4+ cells by simian immunodeficiency virus: productive infection associated with envelope glycoprotein induced fusion. *Proc. Natl Acad. Sci. USA* **86**, 2443–2447.
45. Hattori, T., Koito, A., Takatsuki, K., Kido, H. and Katunuma, N. (1989). Involvement of tryptase-related protease in human immunodeficiency virus type 1 infection. *FEBS* **248**, 48–52.

46. Stephens, P.E., Clements, G., Yokoyama, G.T. and Moore, J. (1990). A chink in HIV's armour? *Nature, Lond.* **343**, 219.

47. Mann, D.L., Lasane, F., Popovic, M. *et al.* (1987). HTLV-III large envelope protein (gp120) suppresses PHA-induced lymphocyte blastogenesis. *J. Immunol.* **138**, 2640–2648.

48. Shalaby, M.R., Krowka, J.F., Gregory, T.J. *et al.* (1987). The effects of human immunodeficiency virus recombinant envelope glycoprotein on immune cell functions *in vitro. Cellular Immunol.* **110**, 140–148.

49. Mittler, R.S. and Hoffmann, M.K. (1989). Synergism between HIV gp120 and gp120 specific antibody in blocking human T cell activation. *Science* **245**, 1380–1382.

50. Gurley, R.J., Ikeuchi, K., Byrn, R.A., Anderson, K. and Groopman, J.E. (1989). CD4+ lymphocyte function with early human immunodeficiency virus infection. *Proc. Natl Acad. Sci. USA* **86**, 1993–1997.

51. Fowlkes, B.J., Schwartz, R.H. and Pardoll, D.M. (1988). Deletion of self reactive thymocytes occurs at a CD4+,8+ precursor stage. *Nature, Lond.* **334**, 620–623.

52. Weinhold, K.J., Lyerly, H.K., Stanley, S.D., Austin, A.A., Matthews, T.J. and Bolognesi, D.P. (1989). HIV-1 gp120-mediated immune suppression and lymphocyte destruction in the absence of viral infection. *J. Immunol.* **142**, 3091–3097.

53. Lanzavecchia, A., Roosnek, E., Gregory, T., Berman, P. and Abrignani, S. (1988). T cells can present antigens such as HIV gp120 targeted to their own surface molecules. *Nature, Lond.* **334**, 530–532.

54. Siliciano, R.F., Lawton, T., Knall, C., Karr, R.W., Gregory, P. and Reinherz, E.L. (1988). Analysis of host–virus interactions in AIDS with anti-gp120 T cell clones: effect of HIV sequence variation and a mechanism for CD4+ cell depletion. *Cell* **54**, 561–575.

55. McCune, J.M., Namikawa, R., Kaneshima, H., Schultz, L.D., Lieberman, M. and Weissman, I.L. (1988). The SCID-hu mouse: murine model for the analysis of human haematolymphoid differentiation and function. *Science* **241**, 1632–1639.

56. Gyorkey, F., Melnick, J.L., Sivikovics, J.G. and Gyorkey, P. (1985). Retrovirus resembling HTLV in macrophages of patients with AIDS. *Lancet* **i**, 106.

57. Vazeux, R., Brousse, N., Jarry, A. *et al.* (1987). AIDS subacute encephalitis: identification of HIV infected cells. *Am. J. Pathol.* **126**, 2360–2364.

58. Michaels, J., Price, R.W. and Rosenblum, M.K. (1988). Microglia in the giant cell encephalitis of acquired immune deficiency syndrome: proliferation, infection and fusion. *Acta Neuropathol.* **76**, 373–379.

59. Patterson, S. and Knight, S. (1987). Susceptibility of human peripheral blood dendritic cells to infection by human immunodeficiency virus. *J. Gen. Virol.* **68**, 1177–1183.

60. Montagnier, L., Gruest, J., Chamaret, S. *et al.* (1984). Adaptation of lymphadenopathy associated virus (LAV) to replication in EBV-transformed B lymphoblastoid cell lines. *Science* **225**, 63–66.

61. Cheng-Mayer, C., Roka, J.T., Rosenblum, M.L., McHugh, T., Stites, D.P. and Levy, J.A. (1987). Human immunodeficiency virus can productively infect cultured human glial cells. *Proc. Natl Acad. Sci. USA* **84**, 3526–3530.

62. Castro, B.A., Cheng-Mayer, C., Evans, L.A. and Levy, J.A. (1989). HIV

heterogeneity and viral pathogenesis. *AIDS (supplement, 1988)* **2**, s17–s28.
63. Dewhurst, S., Bresser, J., Stevenson, M., Sakai, K., Evinger-Hodges, M.J. and Volsky, D.J. (1987). Persistent productive infection of human glial cells by human immunodeficiency virus (HIV) and by molecular clones of HIV. *J. Virol.* **61**, 3774–3782.
64. Clapham, P.R., Weber, J.N., Whitby, D. *et al.* (1989). Soluble CD4 blocks the infectivity of diverse strains of HIV and HIV for T cells and monocytes but not for brain and muscle cells. *Nature, Lond.* **337**, 368–370.
65. Christofinis, G., Papadaki, L., Sattentau, Q.J., Ferns, R.B. and Tedder, R. (1988). HIV replicates in cultured human brain cells. *AIDS* **1**, 229–234.
66. Funke, I., Hahn, A., Rieber, E.P., Weiss, E. and Riethmuller, G. (1987). The cellular receptor (CD4) of the human immunodeficiency virus is expressed on neurons and glial cells in human brain. *J. Exp. Med.* **165**, 1230–1235.
67. Harouse, J.M., Kunsch, C., Hartle, H.T. *et al.* (1989). CD4 independent infection of human neural cells by human immunodeficiency virus type 1. *J. Virol.* **63**, 2527–2533.

4 | Antiretroviral Therapy

DAVID WILKS and ANGUS G. DALGLEISH

Retroviral Research Group, Division of Immunology, Clinical Research Centre, Watford Road, Harrow HA1 3UL, UK

4.1 INTRODUCTION

The management of human retroviral infections can be divided into the treatment of the infectious and neoplastic complications of infection and the prevention of retroviral replication or the elimination of retrovirus-infected cells. This chapter focuses on therapeutic strategies aimed at modifying the underlying viral infection in order to prevent or delay the development of immunodeficiency or neurological deterioration attributed to retroviral infection *per se*.

In spite of the very large number of compounds which have been shown to have antiviral activity against the human immunodeficiency virus (HIV) *in vitro*, only one, zidovudine (3′-azido,3′-deoxythymidine, AZT) has so far been licensed for clinical use, although several others are currently undergoing clinical trials of some form or other [1]. Although promising results obtained in *in vitro* systems led to the speedy development and deployment of AZT, significant clinical toxicity with both AZT and other substances, such as 2′,3′-dideoxycytidine (ddC), has emphasized the need for careful assessment of anti-HIV agents *in vivo*. The prolonged "latency" of HIV infection and the particular characteristics of the patient groups most affected make placebo-controlled, double-blind trials difficult to design within acceptable ethical constraints. Whilst *in vitro* screening of candidate drugs, with clear definition of any possible toxicity, is important, carefully constructed clinical trials must remain the cornerstone of drug assessment.

4.2 SCREENING *IN VITRO* FOR ANTIVIRAL ACTIVITY

Development of new antiviral agents goes hand in hand with basic research into the natural history of infection and viral cell and molecular

AIDS AND THE NEW VIRUSES
ISBN 0–12–200740–9

biology. As knowledge of the mechanisms of virus structure and function grows, so the emphasis in drug development will shift from "random" screening of compounds on the basis of previously observed effects or similarity to established agents, to rational design of compounds intended to interact in predicted ways with elements of the viral life-cycle. Both approaches, however, continue to require *in vitro* screening protocols, particularly in view of the absence of a cheap, widely available and acceptable animal model.

Most screening protocols have the following general characteristics in common:

(1) a cell-based assay system which incorporates all the stages of the viral life-cycle;
(2) a reproducible, quantifiable, virus-mediated effect which may or may not bear a relationship to established *in vivo* pathogenic mechanisms;
(3) a method of establishing the toxicity or otherwise of compounds with antiviral actions at the concentration at which such antiviral effects were seen.

A variety of parameters have been used to quantify virus load and infectivity in tissue culture supernatants, including:

(1) p24 core antigen level;
(2) reverse transcriptase (RT) level;
(3) the capacity of HIV to induce syncytium formation in CD4+ lymphocyte cultures;
(4) immunofluorescent staining of live or fixed cells;
(5) detection of viral DNA by probing Southern blots, with or without amplification by the polymerase chain reaction.

Both p24 and RT levels essentially measure the number of virus particles rather than infectivity [2]. Syncytium induction by HIV constitutes the basis of the syncytium inhibition assay, which has been used as a sensitive, semi-quantitative measure of the antiviral capacity of drugs, antisera and monoclonal antibodies [3, 4].

4.3.1   Syncytium inhibition assay

Supernatant from chronically HIV-infected H9 or CEM cells is serially diluted and added to CD4+ C8166 cells (6×10^3 cells/well). After incubation for one to seven days the wells are examined under low-power light microscopy for the presence of syncytia and the dilution of supernatant that causes syncytia in 50% of wells is determined. This dilution is regarded as the $TCID_{50}$.

Serial dilutions of serum or candidate antiviral agents can be mixed with virus supernatant at a dilution sufficient to give 100 times the previously determined $TCID_{50}$. The wells are scored for the presence of syncytia at 48 h; the lowest concentration of drug or serum that completely inhibits the formation of syncytia is recorded and gives an indication of relative antiviral activity. Other protocols call for the counting of numbers of syncytia to allow calculation of relative percentage inhibitory activity.

This assay may be used to assess neutralization by pre-incubating drugs or antisera with virus containing supernatant, or to assess the capacity of agents to block virus infectivity by reacting with cell surface structures, by pre-incubating the C8166 indicator cells with drugs or antisera before exposing them to virus. AZT inhibits the formation of syncytia in this assay at a concentration of 0.1–1 µg/ml, and infected individuals have type-specific neutralizing antibodies detectable at titres up to 1/1000. Some limited information on cellular toxicity may also be obtained by observation of cell viability in this assay system.

Other screening protocols are based on the quantitative estimation of p24 or RT in culture supernatants determined by commercial or in-house ELISAs. This may be associated with more formal methods of estimating cellular toxicity, for example by incorporating parallel assays assessing cellular protein metabolism and its inhibition by the agent under investigation. The formal *in vitro* determination of cellular toxicity would logically be more extensive, but restricted to those compounds already shown to have antiviral activity at pharmacologically attainable concentrations.

Spickett *et al.* have shown that p24, RT and syncytium inhibition titres do not necessarily correlate one with another [2]. RT activity may persist in culture supernatants for several days after viral replication has ceased. Defective viruses with reduced infectivity may be produced and can give rise to p24 and RT levels comparable with fully infectious forms. Minor modifications to cell culture technique, in particular the use of different concentrations and sources of fetal calf serum in infected and indicator cell cultures, can have profound effects on the results of all three assays. It is important, therefore, that cell culture and assay conditions are rigorously standardized if meaningful and repeatable results are to be obtained.

In the case of compounds that have been designed or deduced to have a specific mechanism of antiviral action, more specific assays may be appropriate. Thus in the case of RT inhibitors, cell free RT inhibition assays have advantages in terms of safety and convenience [5]. Such systems do not, however, present RT in its *in vivo* intracellular context, and thus do not address such issues as cell penetration. A system for the assessment of antiprotease activity has been described by Lambert *et al.* [6]. After exposure of infected cells to putative protease inhibitors, Western blot analysis was performed using monoclonal antibodies against p17, p24 and RT to demonstrate reduced levels of mature *gag/pol* products. Pulse chase experiments were also performed followed by radioimmunoprecipitation using HIV seropositive serum to demonstrate reduced levels of mature proteins and accumulation of *gag* and *gag/pol* precursors.

Screening for possible therapeutic agents to inhibit the high affinity interaction of CD4 with gp120 may, in most instances, be achieved using solid phase or cell-based assays using soluble recombinant CD4 (sCD4) or gp120 (rgp120). Lundin *et al.* have described a specific assay measuring binding of radioiodinated native gp120 to CD4+ cells [7]. This assay may also be performed using labelled recombinant gp120 [8], but care needs to be taken with radioiodination as Chloramine T and Iodogen radioiodination protocols both result in significant loss of antigenicity. Recently an "immunoadhesin" construct bearing the V_1 and V_2 domains of CD4 and the constant region of human IgG_1 heavy chain has been manufactured [9]. This molecule not only has the ability to bind gp120 bivalently and thus with a higher functional affinity even than CD4, but the presence of the Ig heavy chain facilitates attachment of radioactive, fluorescent and enzyme labels and separation of gp120–immunoadhesin complexes by well-established immunological reagents such as Protein A. Whilst the therapeutic potential of this immunoadhesin remains to be demonstrated, it is clearly very useful as a laboratory tool for investigating the CD4–gp120 interaction and for the identification of reagents that interfere with that interaction.

4.3   HIV

The catalogue of the American Fund for AIDS Research lists 86 compounds which are currently undergoing clinical trials in some form or other world-wide [10]. Although even this must be an underestimate, only AZT has to date entered routine clinical practice. Even in the case of AZT, many questions regarding toxicity, efficacy and clinical indications remain unanswered. This review will consider those compounds for which there is at least some evidence of antiviral efficacy.

Figure 4.1 illustrates the viral life-cycle and indicates the points of action of the substances discussed.

4.3.1 Reverse transcriptase inhibitors

(a) *Zidovudine (AZT)*

Viral reverse transcriptase is responsible for the translation of viral RNA to DNA prior to integration of the provirus into the host genome. AZT was the first RT inhibitor to undergo clinical trials and although many other deoxynucleotides have been shown to have equal or better antiviral activity *in vitro*, none has yet successfully completed clinical trials.

The antiretroviral activity of AZT was first reported in 1985 by Mitsuya *et al.* who showed that it could inhibit viral replication *in vitro* at concentrations below 5 μM, at which it did not affect the physiological immunological functions of T and B cells [11]. Phase I trials were reported in the spring of 1986 and the Phase II study, which was prematurely discontinued due to the increased rate of opportunistic infection in the placebo arm, was reported in July 1987 [12, 13].

Pharmacokinetics and actions. AZT is an analogue of thymidine (Figure 4.2), which is phosphorylated by cellular enzymes and, as the 5′-triphosphate, inhibits RT and terminates viral DNA chain elongation. It is absorbed rapidly from the gastrointestinal tract with peak serum concentrations at 1 hour and a bioavailability of 60%. Hepatic metabolism to an inactive and non-toxic metabolite occurs and only 19% of the parent compound is recovered from the urine. Cerebrospinal fluid (CSF) penetration is good with CSF:plasma ratios of 50–100% within 4 h of the first dose [14].

The Phase II study in AIDS and patients with AIDS-related complex (ARC) demonstrated that AZT (250 mg 4 hourly) could reduce mortality and the frequency of opportunistic infections and lead to increased well being, weight gain and a partial reversal of skin anergy in some patients. CD4 counts increased in the treatment group, but declined to pre-treatment levels after 12 weeks in AIDS patients, although not in patients with ARC. There was no significant influence on the incidence of Kaposi's sarcoma (KS). However, it would seem reasonable to attempt to maintain treatment with AZT during treatment for KS, in spite of the combined myelosuppressive effects of AZT, chemotherapeutic agents and interferon. Several groups at the Vth International Conference on AIDS (1989) reported on the success of such combined regimens [15–18].

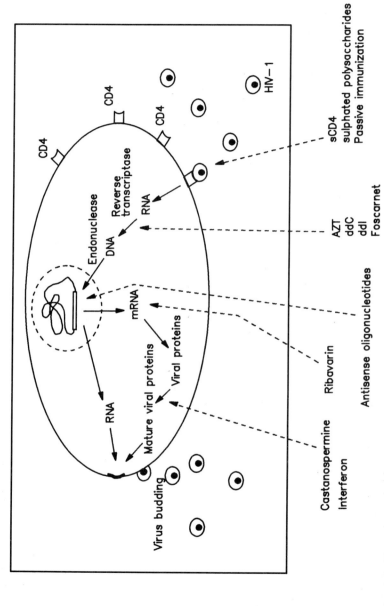

Fig. 4.1   The life-cycle of HIV-1: the points of action of various antiviral agents are indicated (see also Table 4.1).

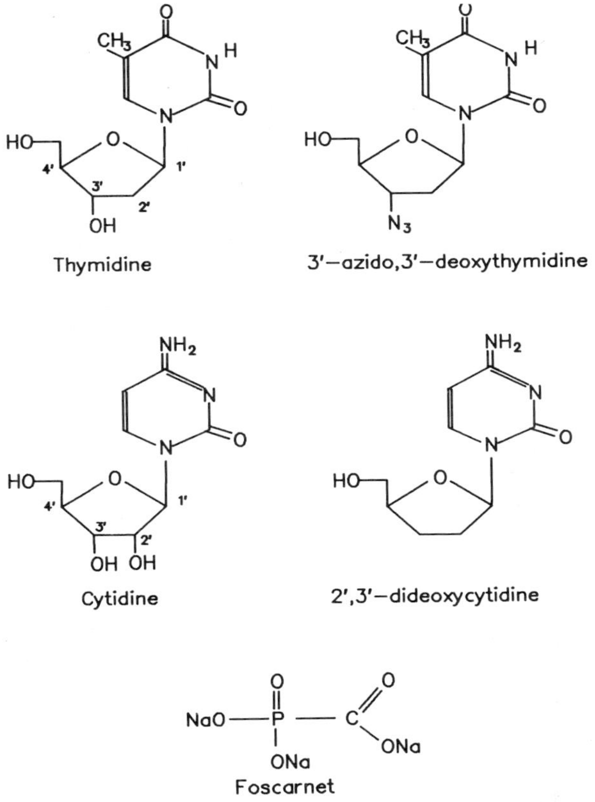

Fig. 4.2 Reverse transcriptase inhibitors: 3′azido,3′-deoxythymidine and 2′,3′-dideoxycytidine are shown with their parent nucleosides.

AZT has been shown to reduce p24 antigenaemia by greater than 90%, even in patients with very high initial levels of p24 [19]. It has also been shown to have beneficial clinical and radiological effects on the neuropsychiatric manifestations of HIV infection [20]. Considerable benefit has been shown in HIV-related thrombocytopenia, and it is now the treatment of choice in this condition in preference to steroids or splenectomy [21, 22].

Toxicity. Significant toxicity, particularly bone marrow depression, was noted during the Phase II study [23]. Nausea, myalgia, insomnia and severe headaches were significantly more common in the treatment group. Anaemia with a haemoglobin count of less than 7.5 g/dl occurred in 24% of the treatment group compared to 4% of placebo recipients. Macrocytosis was also common in the treatment group, although not all of the anaemia seen was macrocytic and macrocytosis was not always associated with anaemia. Neutropenia (<500 cells/mm^3) occurred in 16% of the treatment group compared with 2% of the placebo group. Those patients who entered the trial with low CD4 counts, anaemia, neutropenia or low vitamin B_{12} levels were more likely to suffer myelosuppression. However, B_{12} and folinic acid supplementation have been shown to be of no value in preventing megaloblastic side-effects of AZT [1, 24–26].

Long-term efficacy and AZT resistance.   Two hundred and twenty-nine patients who took part in the original double blind trial were enrolled in an open label follow-up study. The probability of survival at 36 weeks with continuous treatment was higher than would have been expected from previous experience with similar groups of patients (0.92 as opposed to about 0.5). Opportunistic infections occurred, but were less frequent and more amenable to therapy. CD4 counts, which rose with treatment, tended to fall towards baseline levels. Haematological toxicity remained the major adverse reaction. At any given time during the course of the open label study, approximately 50% of the patients were receiving the full dose (200 mg 4 hourly) of AZT, 30% were receiving reduced doses and 20% had temporarily discontinued [27].

In a later dose-ranging study of 74 HIV seropositive individuals with no history of opportunistic infection, haematological side-effects were common but tended to remit after discontinuation of therapy [28, 29]. These side-effects were dose independent in the range 600–1200 mg/day. Skin rashes and pruritis were also seen in 28% of this group. They were less common when AZT was reintroduced after a break in therapy, and have been treated by rapid desensitization [30].

Subsequent experience with much larger patient groups has confirmed this pattern of toxicity and raised the possibility of rarer toxicities including fits. These were not seen in the original study, and since fits occur not infrequently in AIDS patients even in the absence of clinical or radiological evidence of cerebral neoplasia or infection, the significance of their relation to AZT therapy remains to be established.

More unusual side-effects include nail discoloration, affecting 42% of patients in one series, with an increased incidence of black patients [31]. Proximal myopathy occurs in a significant number of patients [32–34]. Myopathy is preceded by a rise in LDH and creatine kinase levels and may necessitate discontinuation of treatment, following which it may resolve.

Prolonged single agent therapy, an immunocompromised host and a virus with a propensity for mutation would seem to be the ideal conditions for the development of resistant strains. Larder *et al.* have isolated strains of HIV-1 that demonstrate *in vitro* AZT resistance from patients on treatment for more than six months [35]. The inhibitory concentration in the assay system used is usually in the region of 0.03 μM, but for resistant strains this figure may be as high as 6 μM. Such strains are more often isolated from sicker patients and duration of therapy is not the only predictor of resistant mutation. Since HIV is not transmitted casually, these resistant mutants do not have the same public health implications as, for example, resistant mycobacteria, but these findings undoubtedly have implications for future treatment protocols, particularly with regard to the treatment of asymptomatic seropositives.

Intermittent and combination AZT regimens. Intermittent therapy with AZT alone for a month followed by a month-long drug-free interval has been reported to reduce the haematalogical side-effects with preservation of beneficial effects on CD4 counts and performance status [36].

AZT has been used in alternate week therapy with 2′,3′-dideoxycytidine (discussed in detail below) and preliminary studies suggest that this regimen reduces the incidence of toxicities attributable to both agents without loss of antiviral effects [37, 38]. It will be important to ascertain whether this strategy also curbs the emergence of resistant strains. AZT-resistant mutants isolated to date remain sensitive to ddC and ddI [35].

AZT has also been used in combination with the established antiherpes virus agent acyclovir [39]. In a pilot study conducted in 1988 of zidovudine in a small group of asymptomatic HIV seropositive individuals, de Wolf *et al.* found significant reductions in p24 levels, but the addition of acyclovir did not result in any additional fall in p24 level [40]. Walger *et al.* suggest that combination therapy of acyclovir and AZT both at 800 mg daily achieves similar benefits to 1200 mg of AZT daily given alone, with a concomitant reduction in side-effects [41].

AZT in asymptomatic infected individuals. The question of the value of AZT therapy in the asymptomatic HIV seropositive individual remains to be answered. Many small uncontrolled trials were reported at Vth International Conference on AIDS (1989), but no large-scale study has yet been completed. Several are in progress world-wide. However, AZT resistance and the high frequency of side-effects suggest that a positive result from these trials is by no means certain. It is interesting to note the experience of Stambuk *et al.* [42]. Of 351 ARC and AIDS patients commenced on AZT, 60% were no longer on treatment after one year, having either died or discontinued treatment due to toxicity.

AZT is a useful drug with undoubted clinical benefits, but whatever the result of large-scale trials, the decision to start treatment in any one case must be made after individual discussion and consideration of the likely risks and benefits to that individual patient.

Other dideoxynucleosides.   Mitsuya and Broder [43] have shown that any purine or pyrimidine with the ribose moiety in a 2',3'-dideoxy configuration has antiviral activity (Fig. 4.2). 2',3'-Dideoxycytidine (ddC) is approximately 10 times more active than AZT against HIV *in vitro* on a molar basis. In a pilot study of ddC (0.03–0.09 mg/kg 4 hourly) given alone, significant increases in CD4 cell counts and reduction in p24 levels were seen. ddC was found to be well absorbed after oral administration and to penetrate the CSF. However severe side-effects were common, in particular a painful peripheral neuropathy which necessitated discontinuation of therapy in all those who took the drug for longer than approximately 10 weeks [37]. Subsequent trials with lower doses of ddC (0.01 mg/kg 4 hourly) have shown reduction of p24 levels in many patients with a much reduced incidence of side-effects. Neuropathy occurred, but was less severe and resolved more quickly after stopping treatment [44].

Other toxicities included rashes, fever, arthralgia, neutropenia and thrombocytopenia. ddC did not, however, cause megaloblastic changes, and in a small associated trial of patients treated with alternating AZT and ddC, each drug taken for a week continuously, side-effects were less common, and treatment could be sustained for up to 18 months in some patients without apparent loss of antiviral effect [38]. Combination therapies may be the key to the effective future use of AZT.

2',3'-Dideoxyinosine (ddI) is another dideoxynucleoside currently under trial. Preliminary reports are promising [45].

(b) *Foscarnet*

Foscarnet (phosphonformate) is a potent non-competitive inhibitor of RT, but it is a highly charged molecule with a short half-life and high intravenous doses are required to achieve therapeutic intracellular levels. A pilot study showed antiviral activity which was lost following discontinuation of therapy [46]. An oral compound has not yet been developed.

(c) *gp120–CD4 interaction*

The high-affinity gp120–CD4 interaction forms the basis of viral tropism for CD4+ cells [4, 47] and is an important site for therapeutic intervention. Soluble constructs of CD4 (sCD4) that lack the transmembrane and cytoplasmic domains have been shown to bind to gp120 with unreduced affinity, to inhibit virus infectivity *in vitro* and to have a beneficial effect on primates infected with simian immunodeficiency virus (SIV$_{mac}$) [48–53]. Although infection of CD4− cells has been demonstrated *in vitro* with difficulty, there is compelling evidence that CD4 functions as the major *in vivo* receptor responsible for infection of lymphocytes and cells of the monocyte/macrophage lineage.

Gp120 has been shown to bind to CD4 at a site that overlaps the site of CD4 for MHC class II binding [54]. Soluble gp120 has been shown to inhibit directly and powerfully the ability of T cell clones to proliferate in response to antigen presented in the context of syngeneic MHC class II [55], and it is possible that blocking of the CD4–class II interaction is responsible for the immunodeficiency of AIDS rather than the direct cytopathic effect of HIV on infected cells [56].

There is no doubt, therefore, that therapeutic agents that block the interaction of CD4 and gp120 would have enormous potential. sCD4 is currently undergoing clinical trials and the results are awaited. Preliminary results suggest that short-term toxicity will not be a problem.

Animal studies suggest that sCD4 will have a short half-life in humans and preliminary studies support this [57]. Recently an "immunoadhesin" bearing the V$_1$ and V$_2$ domains of CD4 spliced to the constant region of an immunoglobulin G$_1$ heavy chain has been manufactured [9]. This molecule has a half-life of 48 h in rabbits. Traunecker *et al.* [58] have reported a similar molecule which bears an IgM constant region and is secreted as a pentamer. This construct is said to have over 1000 times the activity of IgG$_1$ immunoadhesin in the syncytium inhibition assay. The *in vivo* effect of the functional Fc portion of these molecules remains to be determined. It is possible that they may function as neutralizing antibodies contributing to viral clearance or antibody-mediated cellular cytotoxicity (ADCC), but it is also possible that antibody-mediated enhancement of infection may occur. In either case the conserved nature of the CD4 binding site and its necessity in the virus life-cycle suggest that these agents will be active against all infectious isolates and that resistance will not arise through mutation. Clinical trials of both these molecules are awaited.

Anti-idiotype vaccine strategies, which aim to raise antibodies that bear the image of the gp120 binding site on CD4 by immunizing with murine monoclonal antibodies that recognize that site, are also under investigation [59].

(d) *Sulphated polysaccharides*

Sulphated polysaccharides such as dextran sulphate, heparin and pentosan polysulphate are potent antiviral agents *in vitro*. These compounds also possess anticoagulant activity, but this varies between compounds and is not evident at the concentrations at which they exert their antiviral activity [60–62]. They have been shown to protect CD4+ cells from infection *in vitro* at concentrations of 0.1–1 µg/ml, by preventing viral adsorption to cells. Cellular toxicity occurs at concentrations of 2500 µg/ml. Dextran sulphate (DS) is approximately 60 times more active against HIV-2 than HIV-1, and this may be attributed to variations in envelope structure [63]. DS has been shown to induce the regeneration of CD4+ T cells in cultures of lymphocytes from infected individuals, but infected cells are also stimulated to proliferate and there is an associated increase in viral replication [64]. On theoretical grounds, therefore, it seems likely that DS treatment would need to be prescribed in association with drugs that inhibit viral replication.

Clinical trials have been less promising. DS (mol. wt 7000–8000 kD) is poorly absorbed after oral administration, and lower molecular weight forms (e.g. 1000 kD) that might be better absorbed have less antiviral activity [62, 65]. In Phase I dose-ranging studies, oral DS caused alteration of liver function tests, abdominal cramps, bloating and diarrhoea [66]. Studies in mice have shown oral DS to be associated with qualitative and quantitative alterations in bowel flora and sub-total villus atrophy of the intestinal mucosa [67]. Preliminary studies comparing the efficacy of AZT and the combination of AZT with DS in AIDS patients showed no added benefit [68].

(e) *Post-transcriptional processing*

Ribavarin (1-β-ribofuranosyl-1,2,4-triazole carboxamide) has *in vitro* activity against many RNA and DNA viruses. It is a guanosine analogue that interferes with 5' capping of viral mRNA [69]. Early clinical studies suggested that it could reduce the incidence of progression from ARC to AIDS, but this result has not been borne out by further studies [70–72].

HIV *gag* and *gag/pol* proteins undergo considerable post-transcriptional processing before they are functional, and the viral protease would seem to be a good target for therapeutic intervention. No protease inhibitor has yet reached large-scale clinical trials, although early *in vitro* success has been reported using peptides with protease inhibitor activity [6].

Castanospermine (1,6,7,8-tetrahydroxyoctahydroindolizine) is an alkaloid derived from an Australian chestnut tree [73]. *In vitro* it interferes with post-translational glycosylation, inhibiting the cleavage of gp160 to gp120. Synthetic analogues with enhanced *in vitro* antiviral activity have been produced [74].

Avarol is a quinone derivative from the sponge *Dysidea avara*, which inhibits HIV replication *in vitro* by an as yet unknown mechanism. Animal studies have demonstrated low toxicity and good CSF penetration [75]. Human studies of both avarol and castanospermine are awaited.

(f) *Passive immunization*

Vaccination to elicit neutralizing antibodies has classically played an important role in antiviral therapy. The majority of neutralizing anti-envelope antibodies seen in HIV-infected individuals react with immuno-dominant type-specific envelope epitopes, and conserved sites such as the CD4 binding site, tend to be immunosilent [76–78]. In view of the high degree of inter-strain variation, particularly in the *env* gene product, the rapid rate of mutation seen in all retroviruses and the isolation of multiple strains from the same individual at different time points, it seems likely that vaccine strategies will require either to present a cocktail of different strains, or to render immunogenic the conserved, immunosilent regions such as the CD4 binding site [79, 80]. In spite of the above constraints, passive immunization with antiviral antibodies from healthy seropositive donors to infected individuals without antiviral antibodies may be of some value and limited trials have been reported.

Jackson *et al.* [81] have reported the results of transfusing heat-inactivated plasma from asymptomatic donors with high anti-p24 antibodies into patients with AIDS or severe ARC. Improvements were seen in well-being, weight and CD4 counts and p24 antigen levels fell. These effects are said to have persisted for several weeks after treatment. In another uncontrolled study 10 ARC patients received β-propiolactone inactivated plasma from individuals with high-titre antiviral antibodies [82]. No toxicity was reported in individuals receiving plasma from donors of the same ABO group, with some suggestion of benefit to two patients. Hague *et al.* showed that infusion of anti-p24-rich plasma into two children with high levels of circulating p24 and no anti-p24 antibodies resulted in rapid clearance of p24, and stabilization of CD4 cell counts [83].

A fall in anti-p24 antibody levels and a rise in p24 antigen levels is known to predict progression to immunodeficiency [84–86], but whether this results primarily from a reduction in antibody synthesis or an increase in viral replication is not clear. It is evident that passive immunization with anti-p24 antibodies can reduce p24 antigen levels below the limit of detectability, but the fact that p24 levels return to their previous levels six weeks after treatment suggests that infusion has no lasting effect on viral replication and that frequent treatment would be required if this technique were shown to be of any therapeutic value. In view of the logistical problems, type-specific neutralization and the theoretical risk of antibody-dependent enhancement of infection [79, 87], this treatment needs careful and controlled assessment.

(g) *Immunomodulation*

Double-stranded RNAs (dsRNA) promote the production of lympho-kines including tumour necrosis factors (TNF) and interferons (IFN), and have antiviral activity *in vitro*. Ampligen is a dsRNA with periodically mismatched regions (poly(I):poly(C_{12},U)) that has undergone preliminary clinical trials. Twice weekly intravenous injection of 250–500 mg ampligen in 10 patients with AIDS, ARC or persistent generalized lymphadeno-pathy (PGL) resulted in reduction of circulating virus antigen, increases in CD4 counts and improved well-being [88]. Subsequent studies have shown a significant incidence of acute reactions to injection characterized by flushing, diarrhoea, chills and fever. The results of more extensive trials are awaited [89].

Most of the known cytokines that are available in sufficient quantities to be used clinically are currently under trial as immunomodulators. IFN-α has established efficacy in the treatment of KS and reduces viral replication in asymptomatic seropositives [90], although side-effects, such as 'flu-like symptoms, occur in almost all patients. The use of other cytokines remains experimental. Immune activation is known to be a major trigger for viral replication in infected cells [91]; it is therefore likely that any immunostimulatory treatment would need to be combined with drugs that inhibit viral replication. Pilot studies have shown the combination of IL-2 and AZT to be well tolerated [92].

Many other compounds are currently under trial as immunomodulators. The Scandinavian Isoprinosine Study Group (1989) found that isoprino-sine, 3 grams daily given orally, significantly reduced the rate of progression to AIDS in seropositive individuals from 4% to 0.5% over a six-month period of observation, with no serious adverse effects [93]. However, this result was not confirmed by the US/UK Isoprinosine Clinical Investigation, which failed to show any benefit from the drug given at a dose of 4 grams daily. Both of these studies used large numbers of patients (866 and 696, respectively). A smaller study of 50 patients has also failed to show any benefit from isoprinosine [94–96].

(h) *Fusidic acid*

Fusidic acid is a well established antibacterial used predominantly in the treatment of staphylococcal infections. The observation that its use seemed to lead to an improvement in the general condition of an AIDS patient who was being treated for a mycobacterial infection, prompted an investigation of its anti-HIV activity *in vitro*. It was shown to be a potent inhibitor of syncytium formation, albeit at near toxic doses, but a subsequent small clinical trial showed no benefit in 10 patients, illustrating both the importance of *in vivo* studies and the fact that a small well-designed study may rapidly eliminate candidate drugs which turn out to be of no benefit [97, 98].

(i) *AL721*

AL721 is a mixture of lipids which is thought to exert antiviral activity *in vitro* by depleting cell and virion membranes of cholesterol. In a Phase I study of 40 patients taking from 40–100 grams daily, patients gained weight, and mean serum cholesterol levels rose, but no antiviral effect was seen [99]. An important feature of AL721 is the ease with which it is prepared, and many HIV-infected individuals in the UK and the USA already obtain and consume it on a regular basis.

(j) *Antisense oligonucleotides*

Synthetic oligonucleotides of 20–30 base pairs have been investigated for their ability to interfere with viral replication by hybridizing with HIV-specific sequences. Various synthetic backbone derivatives have been used to minimize catabolism by cellular nucleases, and *in vitro* antiviral activity has been recorded. However, many oligonucleotides show *in vitro* activity that is not sequence specific, suggesting that they exert their effect by mechanisms other than specific hybridization. Sequence-specific activity has been reported by Matsukara *et al.* using a 28 base pair phosphorothioate analogue of *rev* [100]. This oligonucleotide is active in infected cell preparations, but there are obvious logistical and pharmacological problems which would need to be overcome to deliver it *in vivo*.

Newer suggested strategies for oligonucleotide approaches include the use of ribozymes: oligonucleotides that mediate self-cleavage and the cleavage of specific target sequences [101]. The delivery of antisense oligonucleotides and ribozymes by retroviral vectors is an interesting option which remains as yet in its infancy.

Table 4.1   Anti-HIV agents.

Site of action	Agents
Prevention of attachment of virus to cell	Soluble CD4 Sulphated polysaccharides Passive immunization
Reverse transcriptase inhibitors	Zidovudine (AZT)[a] 2',3'-dideoxynucleosides,[a] e.g. ddC, ddl Foscarnet
Prevention of transcription of viral DNA and RNA sequences	Antisense oligonucleotides
Inhibition of capping of viral mRNA	Ribavarin
Inhibition of maturation of viral proteins	Castanospermine Interferon
Modulation of host immune response	Ampligen Isoprinosine Miscellaneous cytokines
Cholesterol depletion of viral and host cell membranes	AL721
Unknown	Fusidic acid Avarol

[a] Only these compounds have established clinical efficacy.

(k) *Future clinical trial candidates*

High resolution X-ray crystallography of the tertiary structure of HIV proteinase has confirmed that it belongs to the mechanistic class of aspartic proteinases (102). Detailed analysis of this highly conserved structure should facilitate the rational design of highly specific inhibitors that do not act on cellular proteinases, and which may only consist of short peptides (103). Problems of bioavailability may be overcome by using novel drug delivery systems and clinical trials will probably commence within the next year.

A new class of compounds based on benzodiazepine derivatives (known as TIBO), has been shown to inhibit HIV-1 replication *in vitro*, and has one of the highest therapeutic indices yet reported (104). Examples of these compounds will almost certainly enter clinical trials in the very near future.

4.4 HTLV-I

The treatment of patients known to be seropositive for HTLV-I presents an entirely different situation to HIV. In contrast to HIV, where most if not all infected people may be expected to develop clinical disease within the first decade, only 1–4% of HTLV-I seropositive people will develop adult T cell leukaemia (ATL) or tropical spastic paraparesis (TSP), and these conditions usually develop only after a "latency" of several decades. Thus there is little place for treatment of seropositive individuals who do not have clinical manifestations. Treatment of TSP has not been directed at prevention of viral replication, but rather towards modification of the host immune response. Steroids have been found to be beneficial in two small studies [105, 106]. In a study of 18 patients treated with plasmapheresis, 11 showed significant improvement [107].

4.5 CONCLUSION

One of the most remarkable features of the history of HIV infection during this decade was the rapid deployment of the antiviral AZT, but this drug has now been shown to have several severe side-effects which may limit its usefulness given alone. Many new compounds are under investigation, and it is likely that future AIDS therapies will be multi-drug and multi-modal, within the model already established for cancer therapy.

ADDENDUM

Since this chapter was written there have been a number of developments in the issues discussed, particularly in the use of zidovudine (AZT) in asymptomatic HIV seropositive individuals.

The Multicentre Canadian Azidothymidine Trial [108] reported in September 1989 on the side-effects of AZT in 74 patients belonging to CDC groups IIB, III and IVC2. Symptomatic adverse effects were present in 96% of patients, most commonly nausea (64%), fatigue (55%) and headache (49%). These were generally self-limiting and therapy was only discontinued in three out of 74 patients. Haematological toxicity was common, with megaloblastic changes in 95% of 65 bone marrow specimens after 18 weeks of therapy.

Two major US trials of AZT in early HIV infection were discontinued in August 1989, following preliminary analyses showing reduced progression in AZT-treated patients [109]. In the first trial (ACTG 016), 713 early symptomatic patients with CD4 counts between 200 and 800 cells/µl were allocated to placebo or 1200 mg/day of AZT. At the time of review, 36 placebo patients had progressed to AIDS or "advanced ARC" as opposed to 14 from the treated group. This benefit was shown only in patients whose CD4 counts lay between 200 and 500 cells/µl at entry. Severe toxicity was seen in less than 5% of patients.

In the second trial to be discontinued (ACTG 019), 3200 asymptomatic HIV seropositives were allocated to placebo or either 500 or 1500 mg/day of AZT. Progression to ARC and AIDS in the treatment groups combined was halved with respect to the placebo arm.

It is impossible to interpret these results without the full data, publication of which is still pending. However it is clear that these trials will not now be able to furnish evidence on long-term toxicity of AZT resistance. In view of the high cost of AZT and the high incidence of toxicity, the question of long-term therapy for all asymptomatic seropositives remains unanswered. The MRC/INSERM Concorde I trial, which aims to look at efficacy, toxicity and drug resistance, may provide important information in this respect.

Soluble CD4 and immunoadhesin have both entered early clinical trials but results have not yet been published.

REFERENCES

1. Richman, D.D. (1988). The treatment of HIV infection. *AIDS* **2**, Suppl. 1, S137–S142.
2. Spickett, G., Beattie, R.E., Bountiff, L., Dalgleish, A.G. and Webster, A.D.B. (1989). Quantitation of HIV-1 activity in tissue culture supernatants: effects of culture conditions on syncytial assays and virus production. *J. Virol. Meth.* **24**, 67–76.
3. Popovic, M., Sarngadharan, M.G., Read, E. and Gallo, R.C. (1984). Detection, isolation and continuous production of cytopathic retroviruses (HTLV-III) from patients with AIDS and pre-AIDS. *Science* **224**, 497–500.
4. Dalgleish, A.G., Beverley, P.C.L., Clapham, P.R., Crawford, D.H., Greaves, M.F. and Weiss, R.A. (1984). The CD4(T4) antigen is an essential component of the receptor for the AIDS retrovirus. *Nature, Lond.* **312**, 763.
5. Hoffman, A.D., Banapour, B. and Levy, J.A. (1985). Characterisation of the AIDS associated retrovirus reverse transcriptase and optimal conditions for its detection in virions. *Virology* **147**, 326–335.
6. Lambert, D., Meek, T., Dreyer, G., Leary, J., Metcalf, B. and Pettaway, S.R. (1989). Inhibitors of HIV-1 protease inhibit the processing of gag and gag/pol polyproteins in infected T-cells. *Vth International Conference on*

AIDS, Montreal, June 1989 (Abstract WCO 11).

7. Lundin, K., Nygren, A., Arthur, L.O. *et al.* (1987). A specific assay measuring binding of ^{125}I-gp120 from HIV to T4+/CD4+ cells. *J. Immunol. Meth.* **97**, 93–100.

8. Arthos, J., Deen, K.C., Chaikin, M.A. *et al.* (1989). Identification of the residues in human CD4 critical for the binding of HIV. *Cell* **57**, 469–481.

9. Capon, D.J., Charnow, S.M., Mordenti, J. *et al.* (1989). Designing CD4 immunoadhesins for AIDS therapy. *Nature, Lond.* **337**, 525–531.

10. Abrams, D., Gottlieb, M., Grieco, M. and Speer, M. (1989). *AIDS/HIV Experimental Treatment Directory*, American Foundation for AIDS Research, Vol. 2, No. 4 (February 1989).

11. Mitsuya, H., Weinhold, K.J., Furman, P.A. *et al.* (1985). 3'-azido-3'-deoxythymidine (BWA509U): An antiviral agent that inhibits the infectivity and cytopathic effect of human T-lymphotrophic virus type III/lymphadenopathy-associated virus *in vitro*. *Proc. Natl Acad. Sci. USA* **82**, 7096–7100.

12. Yarchoan, R., Klecker, R.W., Weinhold, K.J. *et al.* (1986). Administration of 3'-azido-3'-deoxythymidine, an inhibitor of HTLV III/LAV replication to patients with AIDS or AIDS-related complex. *Lancet* **i**, 575–580.

13. Fischl, M., Richman, D.D., Grieco, M.H. *et al.* (1987). The efficacy of azidothymidine (AZT) in the treatment of patients with AIDS and AIDS-related complex. *New Engl. J. Med.* **317**, 185–191.

14. Klecker, R.W., Collins, J.M., Yarchoan, R. *et al.* (1987). Plasma and cerebrospinal fluid pharmacokinetics of 3'-azido-3'-deoxythymidine: a novel pyrimidine analog with potential application for the treatment of patients with AIDS and related diseases. *Clin. Pharmacol. Ther.* **41**, 407–412.

15. Fröschl, M., Stallmann, D., Holzmann, H., Landthaler, M. and Braun-Falco, O. (1989). Dermatological manifestations during zidovudine treatment. *Vth International Conference on AIDS*, Montreal, June 1989 (Abstract MBP 365).

16. Gonzalez-Canali, G., Navarro-Carola, E., De Gramont, A., Demuynck, B., Louvet, C. and Krulik, M. (1989). Phase II study of alpha 2A interferon associated with AZT in patients with AIDS related Kaposi's sarcoma. *Vth International Conference on AIDS*, Montreal, June 1989 (Abstract TBP 279).

17. Knechten, H. and Braeck, F. (1989). Remission of Kaposi's sarcoma by a combined therapy with interferon beta and AZT in AIDS patients. *Vth International Conference on AIDS*, Montreal, June 1989 (Abstract TBP 291).

18. Baumann, R. (1989). Combined treatment with zidovudine and lymphoblast interferon alpha in patients with HIV-related Kaposi's sarcoma. *Vth International Conference on AIDS*, Montreal, June 1989 (Abstract WBP 326).

19. Jackson, G.G., Paul, D.A., Falk, L.A. *et al.* (1988). Human Immuno-deficiency Virus (HIV) antigenaemia (p24) in the acquired immuno-deficiency syndrome (AIDS) and the effect of treatment with zidovudine (AZT). *Ann. Int. Med.* **108**, 175–180.

20. Yarchoan, R., Berg, G., Brouwers, P. *et al.* (1987). Response of human immunodeficiency virus associated neurological disease to 3'-azido-3'-

deoxythymidine. *Lancet* **i**, 132–135.
21. Flegg, P.J., Jones, M.E., MacCallum, L.R., Williams, K.G., Cook, M.K. and Brettle, R.P. (1989). Effects of long-term zidovudine on platelet count. *Vth International Conference on AIDS*, Montreal, June 1989 (Abstract TBP 271).
22. Routy, J.P., Blanc, A.P., Garabedian, C., Maurice, C., David, M. and Jolio, Y. (1989). Efficacite de la zidovudine a faible dose dans le traitement des thrombopenies liées au virus HIV. *Vth International Conference on AIDS*, Montreal, June 1989 (Abstract TBP 277).
23. Richman, D.D., Fischl, M., Grieco, M.H. *et al.* (1987). The toxicity of azidothymidine (AZT) in the treatment of patients with AIDS and AIDS-related complex. *New Engl. J. Med.* **317**, 192–197.
24. Clotet, B., Gimeno, J.M., Jou, A., Sirera, G., Tor, J., Dominguez, M. and Foz, M. (1989). Toxicity of zidovudine (AZT) in patients with AIDS. *Vth International Conference on AIDS*, Montreal, June 1989 (Abstract TBP 308).
25. Navarette, M.S., Gharakhanian, S., Cardon, B. and Rozenbaum, W. (1989). Vitamin B12 supplements in patients treated with zidovudine. *Vth International Conference on AIDS*, Montreal, June 1989 (Abstract TBP 307).
26. McCutchen, J.A., Ballard, C., Freeman, B., Bartok, A. and Richman, D. (1989). Cyanocobalamin (Vitamin B12) supplementation does not prevent the haematological toxicity of azidothymidine (AZT). *Vth International Conference on AIDS*, Montreal, June 1989 (Abstract MBP 325).
27. Richman, D.D. and Andrews, J. (1988). Results of continued monitoring of participants in the placebo controlled trial of zidovudine for severe HIV infection. *Am. J. Med.* **85**(2A), 208–213.
28. Fanning, M., Osachoff, J., Montaner, C. *et al.* (1989). Long-term non-haematological adverse effects of AZT and its effect on the pre-treatment symptomatology. *Vth International Conference on AIDS*, Montreal, June 1989 (Abstract WBO 6).
29. Ruedy, J., Montaner, J., Gelmon, K. *et al.* (1989). Nature, time course and dose dependency of zidovudine related side effects. Results from the Multicentre Canadian Azidothymidine Trial (MCAT). *Vth International Conference on AIDS*, Montreal, June 1989 (Abstract MBO 47).
30. MacFadden, D.K. (1989). A method for the rapid desensitisation of patients allergic to AZT. *Vth International Conference on AIDS*, Montreal, June 1989 (Abstract TBP 321).
31. Don, P.C., Fusco, F., Fried, P., Batterman, A., Duncanson, F.P., Lenox, T.H. and Klein, N.C. (1989). Nail dyschromia in zidovudine treated AIDS/ARC patients. *Vth International Conference on AIDS*, Montreal, June 1989 (Abstract MBP 189).
32. Bessen, L.J., Greene, J.B., Louie, E., Seitzman, P. and Weinberg, H. (1988). Severe polymyositis-like syndrome associated with zidovudine treatment of AIDS and ARC. *New Engl. J. Med.* **318**, 708.
33. Fischl, M., Gagnon, S., Uttamchandani, R. *et al.* (1989), Myopathy associated with long term zidovudine therapy. *Vth International Conference on AIDS*, Montreal, June 1989 (Abstract MBP 329).
34. Peters, B., Wilson, G. and Pinching, A.J. (1989). Zidovudine myopathy—a prospective study. *Vth International Conference on AIDS*, Montreal, June

1989 (Abstract MBP 326).

35. Larder, B.A., Darby, G. and Richman, D.D. (1989). HIV with reduced sensitivity to zidovudine (AZT) isolated during prolonged therapy. *Science* **243**, 1731–1734.

36. Staszewski, S., Odewald, J., Gottstein, A., Rehmet, S., Helm, E.B. and Stille, W. (1989). Reduction of zidovudine side effects by an intermittent therapy scheme. *Vth International Conference on AIDS*, Montreal, June 1989 (Abstract WBP 334).

37. Yarchoan, R., Perno, C.F., Thomas, R.V. *et al.* (1988). Phase I studies of 2′,3′-dideoxycytidine in severe human immunodeficiency virus infection as a single agent and alternating with zidovudine (AZT). *Lancet* **i**, 76–81.

38. Yarchoan, R., Pluda, J.M., Thomas, R.V., Perno, C.F., McAtee, N. and Broder, S. (1989). Long term (18 month) treatment of severe HIV infection with an alternating regimen of AZT and 2′,3′-dideoxycytidine (ddC). *Vth International Conference on AIDS*, Montreal, June 1989 (Abstract WBP 327).

39. Surbonne, A., Yarchoan, R., McAtee, N. *et al.* (1988). Therapy of AIDS and AIDS related complex with a regimen of 3′-azido,2′,3′-dideoxythymidine (azidothymidine or zidovudine) and acyclovir. *Ann. Int. Med.* **108**, 534–540.

40. de Wolf, F., Lange, J., Goudsmit, J. *et al.* (1988). Effect of Zidovudine on serum human immunodeficiency virus antigen levels in symptom-free subjects. *Lancet* **i**, 373–376.

41. Walger, P., Baumgart, P., Wilke, G. *et al.* (1989). Effectiveness of low dose combination therapy with azidothymidine (zidovudine) and acyclovir in AIDS and ARC patients. *Vth International Conference on AIDS*, Montreal, June 1989 (Abstract WBP 318).

42. Stambuk, D., Mir, N., Hawkins, D., Costello, C. and Gazzard, B. (1989). The toxicity of zidovudine in the treatment of patients with AIDS related complex and AIDS. *Vth International Conference on AIDS*, Montreal, June 1989 (Abstract TBP 326).

43. Mitsuya, H. and Broder, S. (1986). Inhibition of the in vitro infectivity and cytopathic effect of human T-lymphotrophic virus type III/lymphadeno-pathy associated virus (HTLV-III/LAV) by 2′,3′-dideoxynucleosides. *Proc. Natl Acad. Sci. USA* **83**, 1911–1915.

44. Gottlieb, M., Galpin, J., Thompkins, J., Wilson, D., Donatacci, L. and Soo, W. (1989). 2′,3′-dideoxycytidine (ddC) in the treatment of patients with AIDS and ARC. *Vth International Conference on AIDS*, Montreal, June 1989 (Abstract ThBO 3).

45. Yarchoan, R., Thomas, R.V., Pluda, J.M. *et al.* (1989). Escalating dose phase I study of intravenous and oral 2′,3′-dideoxyinosine (ddI) in patients with AIDS or ARC. *Vth International Conference on AIDS*, Montreal, June 1989 (Abstract ThBO 4).

46. Farthing, C.F., Dalgleish, A.G., Clark, A. *et al.* (1987). Phosphonformate (foscarnet): a pilot study in AIDS and the AIDS related complex. *AIDS* **1**, 21–25.

47. Klatzmann, D., Champagne, E., Chamart, S. *et al.* (1984). T-lymphocyte T4 molecule behaves as the receptor for human retrovirus LAV. *Nature, Lond.* **312**, 767.

48. Deen, K.C., McDougal, J.S., Inacker, R. *et al.* (1988). A soluble form of

CD4(T4) protein inhibits AIDS virus infection. *Nature, Lond.* **331**, 82–84.
49. Fisher, R.A., Bertonis, J.M., Meier, W. *et al.* (1988). HIV infection is blocked *in vitro* by recombinant soluble CD4. *Nature, Lond.* **331**, 76–78.
50. Hussey, R.E., Richardson, N.E., Kowalski, M. *et al.* (1988). A soluble CD4 protein selectively inhibits HIV replication and syncytium formation. *Nature, Lond.* **331**, 78–81.
51. Smith, D.H., Byrn, R.A., Marsters, S.A., Gregory, T., Groopman, J.E. and Capon, D.J. (1987). Blocking of HIV-1 infectivity by a soluble secreted form of the CD4 antigen. *Science* **238**, 1704.
52. Traunecker, A., Luke, W. and Karjalainen, K. (1988). Soluble CD4 molecules neutralise human immunodeficiency virus type 1. *Nature, Lond.* **331**, 84–86.
53. Letvin, N.L., Watanabe, M., Reimann, K.A., Delong, P.A., Liu, T. and Fisher, R.A. (1989). Effect of recombinant soluble CD4 in rhesus monkeys infected with simian immunodeficiency virus of macaques. *Vth International Conference on AIDS*, Montreal, June 1989 (Abstract ThCO 16).
54. Clayton, L.K., Sieh, M., Pious, D.A. and Reinherz, E.L. (1989). Identification of human CD4 residues affecting class II MHC versus HIV-1 gp120 binding. *Nature, Lond.* **339**, 548–551.
55. Manca, F., Habeshaw, J.A. and Dalgleish, A.G. (1990). HIV envelope glycoprotein inhibits antigen specific T cell responses and is blocked by soluble CD4. *Lancet* **335**, 811–815.
56. Habeshaw, J.A. and Dalgleish, A.G. (1989). The relevance of the HIV env/CD4 interaction to the pathogenesis of the acquired immuno-deficiency syndrome. *J. AIDS* **2**, 457–468.
57. Kahn, J., Davis, A.J., Groopman, J., Kaplan, L., Sherwin, S. and Volbeording, P. (1989). Pharmacokinetic studies of recombinant soluble CD4 in patients with AIDS and AIDS-related complex. *Vth International Conference on AIDS*, Montreal, June 1989 (Abstract ThBO 5).
58. Traunecker, A., Schneider, J., Keifer, H. and Karjalainen, K. (1989). Highly efficient neutralization of HIV with recombinant CD4-immunoglobulin molecule. *Nature, Lond.* **339**, 68–70.
59. Dalgleish, A.G., Thomson, B.J., Chanh, T.C., Malkovsky, M. and Kennedy, R.C. (1987). Neutralisation of HIV isolates by anti-idiotypic antibodies which mimic the T4(CD4) epitope: a potential AIDS vaccine. *Lancet* **ii**, 1047.
60. Ueno, R. and Kuno, S. (1987). Dextran sulphate, a potent anti-HIV agent *in vitro* having synergism with zidovudine. *Lancet* **i**, 1379.
61. Nakashima, H., Kido, Y., Kobayashi, N., Motoki, Y., Neushul, M. and Yamamoto, N. (1987). Purification and characterization of an avian myeloblastosis and human immunodeficiency virus reverse transcriptase inhibitor: sulfated polysaccharides extracted from sea algae. *Antimicrob. Agents Chemother.* **31**, 1524–1528.
62. De Clercq, E. (1989). Potential drugs for the treatment of AIDS. *J. Antimicrob. Chemother.* **23**, 35–46.
63. Pauwels, R., Baba, M., Schols, D., Balzarini, J., Desmyter, J. and De Clercq, E. (1989). Differential anti-retroviral activity of dextran sulfate, pentosan polysulfate and heparin against HIV-1 (HTLV-IIIB) and HIV-2 (LAV-2 ROD). *Vth International Conference on AIDS*, Montreal, June

1989 (Abstract C595).

64. Izaguirre, C.A. and Drouin, J. (1989). The anti-HIV drugs castanospermine and dextran sulfate allow the growth of *in vivo* infected CD4+ T cells. *Vth International Conference on AIDS*, Montreal, June 1989 (Abstract ThBO 48).

65. Baba, M., Schols, D., Pauwels, R., Nakashima, H., Balzarini, J. and De Clercq, E. (1989). Comparative inhibitory effects of sulfated polysaccharides on giant cell formation induced by co-cultivation of CD4+ cells with persistently HIV-1-infected cells. *Vth International Conference on AIDS*, Montreal, June 1989 (Abstract MCP 75).

66. Abrams, D., Pettinelli, C., Power, M., Kubacki, V.B., Grieco, M.H. and Henry, W.K. (1989). A phase I/II dose ranging trial of oral dextran sulfate in HIV p24 antigen positive individuals (ACTG 060); results of a safety and efficacy trial. *Vth International Conference on AIDS*, Montreal, June 1989 (Abstract WBP 315).

67. Wells, C.L., Erlandsen, S.L. and Rhame, F.S. (1989). Effect of oral dextran sulfate on the mouse intestine. *Vth International Conference on AIDS*, Montreal, June 1989 (Abstract WBP 289).

68. Brockmeyer, N.H., Mertins, L. and Goos, M. (1989). Effect of a combined dextrane sulfate/zidovudine therapy compared to zidovudine monotherapy in AIDS. *Vth International Conference on AIDS*, Montreal, June 1989 (Abstract WBP 324).

69. Goswami, B.B., Borek, E. and Sharma, O. (1979). The broad spectrum antiviral agent ribavarin inhibits capping of RNA. *Biochem. Biophys. Res. Commun.* **89**, 830–836.

70. Roberts, R.B., Makuch, R. and Jurica, K. (1989). Phase I trial of oral ribavarin in high risk patients for AIDS. *Vth International Conference on AIDS*, Montreal, June 1989 (Abstract ThBO 1).

71. Schulof, R., Simon, G., Parenti, D. *et al.* (1989). Phase I/II trial of ribavarin and isoprinosine in asymptomatic HIV viraemic gay men. *Vth International Conference on AIDS*, Montreal, June 1989 (Abstract ThBO 2).

72. Spanish Ribavarin Study Group (1989). Comparison of ribavarin versus placebo for preventing the progression of HIV infected subjects from CDC stage III to stage IV. *Vth International Conference on AIDS*, Montreal, June 1989 (Abstract TBP 294).

73. Clumeck, N. and Hermans, P. (1988). Antiviral drugs other than zidovudine and immunomodulating therapies in human immunodeficiency virus infection. *Am. J. Med.* **85**, 165–172.

74. Sunkara, P.S., Taylor, D., Kang, M. *et al.* (1989). Castanospermine analogs as potent inhibitors of HIV. *Vth International Conference on AIDS*, Montreal, June 1989 (Abstract MCP 117).

75. Sarin, P.S. (1988). Molecular pharmacologic approaches to the treatment of AIDS. *Ann. Rev. Pharmacol.* **28**, 411–428.

76. Robert-Guroff, M., Brown, M. and Gallo, R.C. (1985). HTLV-III neutralising antibodies in patients with AIDS and AIDS-related complex. *Nature, Lond.* **316**, 72.

77. Weiss, R.A., Clapham, P.R., Chiengsong-Popov, R. *et al.* (1985). Neutralisation of human T-lymphotropic virus type III by sera of AIDS and AIDS-risk patients. *Nature, Lond.* **316**, 69.

78. Weiss, R.A., Clapham, P.R., Weber, J.N., Dalgleish, A.G., Lasky, L.A.

and Berman, P.W. (1986). Variable and conserved neutralisation antigens of the human immunodeficiency virus. *Nature, Lond.* **324**, 572.

79. Cheng-Mayer, C., Homsy, J., Evans, L.A. and Levy, J.A. (1988). Identification of human immunodeficiency virus subtypes with distinct patterns of sensitivity to serum neutralisation. *Proc. Natl Acad. Sci. USA* **85**, 2815–2819.

80. Hahn, B.H., Shaw, G.M., Taylor, M.E. *et al.* (1986). Genetic variation in HTLV-III/LAV over time in patients with AIDS or at risk for AIDS. *Science* **232**, 1548–1553.

81. Jackson, G.G., Perkins, J.T., Rubenis, M. *et al.* (1988). Passive immuno-neutralization of human immunodeficiency virus in patients with advanced AIDS. *Lancet* **ii**, 647–652.

82. Karpas, A., Hill, F., Youle, M. *et al.* (1989). Effects of passive immunization in patients with the acquired immunodeficiency syndrome-related complex and acquired immunodeficiency syndrome. *Proc. Natl Acad. Sci. USA* **85**, 9234–9237.

83. Hague, R., Yap, P.L., Mok, J.Y.Q., Jackson, G.G., Hargreaves, F.D. and Coutts, N.A. (1989). Infusion of anti p24 antibody rich plasma in two children with persistent HIV antigenaemia. *Vth International Conference on AIDS*, Montreal, June 1989 (Abstract TBP 246).

84. Lange, J.M., Paul, D.A., Huisman, H.G. *et al.* (1986). Persistent HIV antigenaemia and decline of HIV core antibodies associated with transition to AIDS. *Br. Med. J.* **293**, 1459–1462.

85. Lange, J.M. and Goudsmit, J. (1987). Decline of antibody reactivity to HIV core protein secondary to increased production of HIV antigen. *Lancet* **i**, 448.

86. Weber, J.N., Clapham, P.R., Weiss, R.A. *et al.* (1987). Human immuno-deficiency virus infection in two cohorts of homosexual men: neutralising sera and association of anti-gag antibody with prognosis. *Lancet* **i**, 119–122.

87. Robinson, W.E., Montefiori, D.C. and Mitchell, W.M. (1988). Antibody dependent enhancement of human immunodeficiency virus type 1 infection. *Lancet* **i**, 790–794.

88. Carter, W.A., Strayer, D.R., Brodsky, I. *et al.* (1987). Clinical immuno-logical and virological effects of ampligen, a mismatched double stranded RNA in patients with AIDS or AIDS-related complex. *Lancet* **i**, 1286–1292.

89. Pazin, G.J., Huang, X.L., McMahon, D. *et al.* (1989). Acute responses to ampligen infusions in HIV-infected people. *Vth International Conference on AIDS*, Montreal, June 1989 (Abstract WBP 303).

90. Davey, V., Kovacs, J.A., Herpin, B. *et al.* (1989). A placebo controlled trial of interferon alfa-2B in asymptomatic HIV infection. *Vth International Conference on AIDS*, Montreal, June 1989 (Abstract ThBO 43).

91. Folks, T.M., Justement, J., Kinter, A. *et al.* (1987). Cytokine induced expression of HIV-1 in a chronically infected promonocyte cell line. *Science* **238**, 800–802.

92. Bartlett, J.A., Blankenship, K.D., Greenberg, M. *et al.* (1989). The safety of zidovudine and interleukin-2 in asymptomatic HIV infected patients. *Vth International Conference on AIDS*, Montreal, June 1989 (Abstract WBP 325).

93. Scandinavian Isoprinosine Study Group (1989). Isoprinosine reduced clinical progression in HIV infected patients in a double blind placebo controlled trial. *Vth International Conference on AIDS*, Montreal, June 1989 (Abstract ThBO 46).

94. Bekesi, J.G., Tsang, P.H., Wallace, J.I. and Roboz, J.P. (1987). Immunorestorative properties of isoprinosine in the treatment of patients at high risk of developing ARC or AIDS. *J. Clin. Lab. Immunol.* **24**, 155–161.

95. Loveless, M.O., Robins, D.S. *et al.* (1989). The effect of isoprinosine R (inosine prabonex) in HIV seropositive patients with a low risk for developing AIDS. *Vth International Conference on AIDS*, Montreal, June 1989 (Abstract WBP 288).

96. Barbaro, D. and Fragua, H. (1989). Failure of isoprinosine in prevention of ARC to AIDS. *Vth International Conference on AIDS*, Montreal, June 1989 (Abstract WBP 304).

97. Faber, V., Dalgleish, A.G., Newell, A. and Malkovsky, M. (1987). Inhibition of HIV replication *in vitro* by fusidic acid. *Lancet* **ii**, 827–828.

98. Youle, M.S., Hawkins, D.A., Lawrence, A.G. *et al.* (1989). Clinical, immunological and virological effects of sodium fusidate in patients with the acquired immunodeficiency syndrome or AIDS related complex: an open study. *J. AIDS* **2**, 59–62.

99. Mildvan, D., Armstrong, D., Antoniskis, D. *et al.* (1989). An open label dose-ranging trial of AL721 in PGL and ARC. *Vth International Conference on AIDS*, Montreal, June 1989 (Abstract WBP 312).

100. Matsukara, M., Shinozuka, K., Zon, G., Mitsuya, H., Reitz, M., Cohen, J.S. and Broder, S. (1987). Phosphorthioate analogs of oligodeoxy-nucleotides: inhibitors of replication and cytopathic effects of HIV. *Proc. Natl Acad. Sci. USA* **84**, 7706–7710.

101. Sarver, N., McGowan, J. and Johnston, M.I. (1989). Potential of autocatalytic self-cleaving RNAs as anti-HIV agents. *Vth International Conference on AIDS*, Montreal, June 1989 (Abstract MCP 58).

102. Lapatto, R., Blundell, T., Hemmings, A. *et al.* (1989). X-ray analysis of HIV-1 proteinase at 2.7 A resolution confirms structural homology among retroviral enzymes. *Nature, Lond.* **342**, 299–302.

103. Roberts, N.A., Martin, J.A., Kinchington, D. *et al.* (1990). Rational design of peptide-based HIV proteinase inhibitors. *Science* **248**, 358–361.

104. Pauwels, R., Andries, K., Desmyter, J. *et al.* (1990). Potent and selective inhibition of HIV-1 replication *in vitro* by a novel series of TIBO derivatives. *Nature, Lond.* **343**, 470–474.

105. Osame, M., Matsumoto, M., Usuku, K. *et al.* (1987). Chronic progressive myelopathy associated with elevated antibodies to human T-lymphotrophic virus type I and adult T-cell leukaemia like cells. *Ann. Neurol.* **21**, 117–122.

106. Cruikshank, K., Rudge, P., Dalgleish, A.G. *et al.* (1989). Tropical spastic paraparesis and human T cell lymphotrophic virus type 1 in the United Kingdom. *Brain* **112**, 1057–1090.

107. Matsuo, H., Nakamura, T., Tsujihata, M. *et al.* (1988). Plasmapheresis in the treatment of human T-cell lymphotrophic virus type 1 associated myelopathy. *Lancet* **ii**, 1109–1113.

108. Gelmon, K., Montaner, J.S.G., Fanning, M. *et al.* (1989). Nature, time

course and dose dependence of zidovudine-related side effects: results from the Multicenter Canadian Azidothymidine Trial. *AIDS* **3**, 555–561.

109. Editorial. Clinical trials of zidovudine in HIV infection. (1989). *Lancet* **ii**, 483–484.

5 | Strategies in the Quest for an HIV Vaccine

GORDON L. ADA

Department of Immunology and Infectious Diseases, Johns Hopkins School of Hygiene and Public Health, Baltimore, MD 21205, USA

5.1 INTRODUCTION

AIDS has now assumed the characteristics of a world pandemic with cases reported from the great majority of countries in the world. Rarely, if ever, has so much effort been directed towards elucidating the properties of the causative agent, the human immunodeficiency virus (HIV), the nature of the immune response generated in infected people, the progressive deterioration of the immune process, the symptoms of disease which appears some years after infection of most people and the events which result in death of infected people. Parallel with these observations is the widespread effort being made by major sections of the scientific/medical community to find means of prevention and/or alleviation of these symptoms. Because of the nature of the virus, its mode of replication, the range of cells susceptible to infection and the mode of transmission, the view is commonly expressed that for the near future at least, a combination of treatments may be required to prevent or control infections. Some are simple in theory, e.g. use of condoms or changes in personal life-style, but require substantial modifications to social behaviour which are generally not easy to achieve. Others are expensive, such as treatment with drugs. The countries at greatest risk of deterioration of social patterns and health welfare are in the least developed category, and particularly many are in Africa. Many of the newly developed approaches to treatment will be out of the reach of the majority of affected people.

Judged on past public health experience, the availability of an effective and inexpensive vaccine is the most cost-effective procedure for control of infectious disease. Unfortunately, HIV has many attributes which contribute to the difficulty of developing an effective vaccine [1, 2]. As the pool of information on new developments increases, however, this allows fresh perspectives, so that these difficulties can be reconsidered.

This chapter examines recent findings and developments concerning

AIDS AND THE NEW VIRUSES
ISBN 0–12–200740–9

HIV-1. The first section reviews and comments upon several aspects relevant to vaccination in general. The events that occur during HIV infection are then discussed with respect to these points, before going on to consider future possibilities.

5.2   EXPECTATIONS OF A VACCINE TO PREVENT/CONTROL INFECTION

Vaccination is only one of many forms of immunotherapy. It can be defined as a process of immunization involving one or a few administrations of the immunogen which should result in long-lasting immunity or protection from disease caused by the pathogen. Immunization is usually carried out at any time — for a short or a long period — *before* exposure to the natural pathogen occurs. It therefore primarily involves the adaptive component of the immune response, even though immunization may be at a site where natural infection also occurs and therefore might stimulate local non-specific immunity. There is no reason to believe that the effect of the latter would persist for extended periods. Already infected people may also be deliberately immunized, e.g. with rabies vaccine. In this situation, elicited non-adaptive responses might play a role in control of the infection.

Vaccination therefore mainly involves T and B cell activation. As effector forms of both cell types generally have short half-lives, vaccination, to be effective in the long term, should achieve two goals:

(1) the generation of large numbers of memory T and B lymphocytes;
(2) the persistence of antigen (or an equivalent situation — see below) in such a form and at an appropriate site so that there is continuing recruitment of the B memory cells to form antibody-secreting cells (ASCs) [3, 4].

Despite great advances in knowledge and understanding of many aspects of immunology in recent years, there are several gaps and one of these is the pathways leading to memory T and B cell generation [1]. Generally, memory cell generation seems to be less demanding than effector cell generation, as illustrated by several demonstrations that two or more serial injections of "sub-immunogenic" aliquots of antigen can lead to an enhanced antibody responses.

Non-infectious antigen is known to persist for very long periods of time in an immunologically relevant form of follicular dendritic cells in lymphoid tissues [5, 6] and there is considerable evidence that antigen so localized may effectively stimulate memory B cells [7]. It has also been postulated that idiotype–anti-idiotype responses may be important in maintenance of long-lived antibody responses [8].

5.3 ROLE OF SPECIFIC ANTIBODY IN INFECTIOUS PROCESSES

Specific antibody has long been considered the immune response of greatest importance in the design of vaccines. It may serve several functions, as described below.

5.3.1 Neutralization of infectivity of the agent

There are examples from all types of infectious agents where antibody specific for a surface component of the agent may prevent infection. Viruses provide the greatest number of examples where such antigens have been detected and analysed, with the following conclusions:

(1) usually one surface antigen is immunodominant for neutralization, e.g. the haemagglutinin (HA) of influenza virus;
(2) neutralizing antibodies react with certain regions (sequences) of the molecules only. These are often hydrophilic and show enhanced atomic mobility, i.e. there is room for atoms to move [9];
(3) where the surface of the agent displays a mosaic of identical molecules, e.g. HA trimers of influenza virua, or 60mers of VP1 in polio virus, neutralizing antibodies frequently recognize tertiary or quaternary shapes, contributed by discontinuous sequences [10]. At present, there is no certain procedure for mimicking such patterns using synthetic peptides which will be immunogenic.

5.3.2 Blocking antibody

Some infectious agents, particularly viruses, and in the absence of neutralizing antibody, only infect cells bearing specific receptors. Antibody to such receptors may block infection, at least *in vitro* [11]. To the author's knowledge, this approach has not yet been shown completely to prevent infection *in vivo*, e.g. the work with rhinovirus [12]. Antiviral antibody may also block the fusion between viral envelope and the cell plasma membrane.

In the absence of neutralizing or blocking antibody (or possibly of very high levels of a factor such as interferon, which would not normally be present in an immunized host prior to exposure to the infectious agent), infection will occur. However, antibody may also be useful in aiding the control of the infection, once established.

5.3.3   Antibody-dependent cellular cytotoxicity (ADCC)

Killer cells which bear Fc receptors may attach to antibody bound to infected cells expressing on their surface antigens of the infectious agent. The exact lineage of these cells is uncertain, but the action of the cells is not MHC-antigen restricted.

5.3.4   Complement-dependent lysis of infected cells

If specific antibody of an appropriate isotype is present and the infected cells express receptors, a "membrane attack complex" may be formed, which results in lysis of the cell.

There are many *in vitro* examples which attest to the efficacy of these two mechanisms in reducing viral titres, but there seem to be few examples showing their effectiveness in clearing an infection *in vivo* in the absence of an effector T cell response. This author is unaware of any experiments which demonstrate complete clearance of an infectious organism in the presence of specific antibody, but in the absence of effector T cells. Furthermore, it is well known that agammaglobulinaemic people survive viral infections such as influenza.

5.4   ROLE OF SPECIFIC T CELL RESPONSES IN THE INFECTIOUS PROCESS

In contrast to the recognition of antigen by specific immunoglobulin receptors on B cells, T cells — both class I and II restricted responses — recognize antigen which has been "processed" by the antigen-presenting cell (APC). This processing results in the formation of peptides which associate with MHC molecules and the complex is transported to the APC plasma membrane [13, 14]. The T cell receptor, like the B cell immunoglobulin receptor, recognizes the tertiary conformation of the complex of which the antigenic peptide is only a part.

This process of T cell activation has several important consequences, including:

(1) T cell responses are classified as MHC class I or II restricted responses, according to the receptor specificity of the T cell. Class I

cells have the CD8 marker, and class II cells, the CD4 marker. Generally, but *not absolutely*, the two classes of T cells have different activities — class II cells mediate help (Th) or delayed-type hypersensitivity (Td) responses, and class I cells mediate cytotoxic (Tc) and suppressor (Ts) activities. Though the pathways of recognition by and activation of Th, Td and Tc are known, similar information for Ts is lacking.

(2) T cell responses are only generated after antigenic peptides are formed, i.e. after infection has occurred. This in effect means that effector T cells, both as regulators (Th and Ts) and effectors (Tc and Ts) will be involved in *controlling or clearing*, as distinct from *preventing*, infections.

(3) In contrast to neutralizing antibody, which reacts with a few epitopes on only one or sometimes two viral proteins, *all proteins* of an infectious agent, in principle, may contribute antigenic peptides that may bind to MHC antigens. In those cases where it has now been studied, such as in influenza and lymphocytic choriomeningitis viruses, "internal" antigens, such as the nucleoprotein that are not recognized by neutralizing antibody, are major contributors of these peptides. Generally, internal antigens show little if any antigenic variation. This means that if a virus showing antigenic drift in surface antigens escapes neutralization by antibody, the T cell response (particularly Tc cells) will in effect be cross-reactive and hence cross-protective.

There is a large body of evidence in model systems that infection by many viruses induces the generation of specific MHC-class I restricted T cells showing cytolytic activity *in vitro* [15]. In many cases it has been shown that these cells, upon transfer, can clear the viral infection. This has been demonstrated with primary (uncultured) cells, with secondary (short-term culture, e.g. 6 days) and with cloned T cells. Cultured or cloned preparations of class II restricted cells may also have cytolytic activity *in vitro* [16–18]. In some systems, transfer of class II restricted human T cells may enhance immunopathological effects (see below). Such findings have raised the possibility that *in vivo*, apart from possible cytolytic activity [19], effector T cells mediate activities largely through secretion of specific lymphokines, such as IFN-γ. A great variety of factors, generally termed cytokines, are now well documented and many have been produced for experimental purposes using recombinant DNA technology.

5.5   PROPERTIES OF HIV RELEVANT TO VACCINE DEVELOPMENT

5.5.1   Structure of the virus

All retrovirus genomes have certain characteristics, including regulatory sequences present at either end of the DNA provirus, long terminal repeats (LTRs), and genes encoding viral proteins that have structural or enzymatic properties. The HIV genome is now recognized to be more complicated in this respect than previously studied retroviruses. A recent map of the organization of the HIV genome is shown in Fig. 5.1 and is described below. The LTRs contain regulatory segments important for viral replication.

Seven proteins are encoded by the HIV-1 genome — *gag*, *pol*, A, *tat*, *env*, B and *art/trs*. The *gag* gene encodes the "group-specific antigens" and is translated as a polyprotein precursor molecule, p55, which is cleaved to form at least three products as illustrated (Fig. 5.1). The products of the *pol* gene have enzymatic activities — a reverse transcriptase (p51 or p66), an endonuclease (p31) and a protease (p10). The precise function of the A (*sor* or Q) gene, p23, is unknown, other than a role in the structure of the infectious virion. The *tat* protein, p14, is encoded by an mRNA containing two exons, located as illustrated in Fig. 5.1, and functions as a potent *trans* activator of HIV expression. The *art/trs* protein, p19, also has a viral regulatory function, being required for the processing and translation of *gag* and *env* RNAs. The B (F or 3' *orf*) protein, p27, located as shown in Fig. 5.1, may act as a negative regulator of viral replication. The envelope protein, *env* or gp160, is processed to form two envelope glycoproteins, gp120 and gp41. In the virion the major glycoprotein, gp120, is attached to the transmembrane protein, gp41, but during isolation of virions gp120 is variably shed. The major properties and functions of these two proteins will be described later.

The LTRs and the regulatory functions of the different proteins described above will not be discussed here further except to comment that should at any stage an attenuated or genetically modified, live viral preparation be considered as the basis of a vaccine, the status (e.g. absence, modification, etc.) of such elements would need to be well defined.

5.5.2   The process of infection by HIV

Cells susceptible to viral infection possess a specific receptor, which for HIV, was shown to be the CD4 molecule [20, 21]. This molecule is a

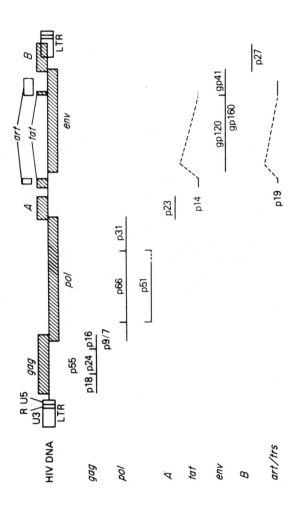

Fig. 5.1 HIV genomic organization. The location of the viral LTRs and coding sequences are shown. The entire HIV proviral genome is 9.7 kb in length. Reprinted from Rabson [27], p. 236, by courtesy of Marcel Dekker, Inc.

major T cell marker, being involved in the specific interaction between the T cell and the antigen-presenting cell. It is, however, now known to be present on a wide variety of cells [22], including macrophages, monocytes and astrocytes. Anti-CD4 antibodies block infection of cells by HIV in tissue culture [20, 21], as can soluble CD4 [23]. However, it became doubtful whether all cells from which HIV has been recovered express CD4 [22] and it has now been shown that neither soluble CD4 nor anti-CD4 antibodies inhibit infection of glioma and rhabdomyosarcoma cells [24]. The mechanism of entry into these cells is at present unknown. Options include a separate, distinct receptor; uptake of virus–antibody complexes; phagocytosis/pinocytosis. The cell lines used in this recent study may not be representative of the situation *in vivo*. Although administration of soluble CD4 to monkeys infected with simian immunodeficiency virus (SIV) has been shown to have a marked therapeutic effect on the disease process [25], this therapy has so far not cured the infection.

Other means by which HIV might enter cells such as macrophages and monocytes is through interaction of complexes containing virus and antibody and/or complement binding to cells which possess receptors for Fc (FcR) or for complement (CR).

However, as mere possession of the CD4 molecule by a cell does not mean susceptibility to infection (murine cells transfected with DNA coding for CD4 are not susceptible to infection by HIV-1), other events such as fusion of the virus with the cell plasma membrane are involved. Interaction between a fusogenic segment of gp41 with the cell membrane results in fusion of the viral envelope with the membrane in a pH-independent process [26].

Once internalized, the viral RNA genome undergoes reverse transcriptase leading first to single-stranded and then double-stranded forms of DNA. Some of the dsDNA is integrated into the host cell genome via the virally coded endonuclease. The DNA provirus undergoes transcription to generate progeny virion RNA and mRNA. Translation of the mRNA yields the various viral proteins [27]. Two aspects of this replication cycle are of particular importance from the point of view of vaccine development:

(1) The virus may persist as a latent infection (as a provirus) without expression of viral antigens and thus presumably escape immune processes.

(2) A high rate of mutation may occur in each of the three steps in the replication process mentioned above because of the lack of error-correcting mechanisms at each step [28]. Though many of the

mutations are most likely lethal for the virus, others are thought to contribute to the great antigenic variation seen in the *env* protein, as discussed later.

5.5.3 The pattern of infection by HIV *in vivo*

(a) *Transmission*

HIV is transmitted by four main processes:

(1) by anal and/or vaginal sexual intercourse, the importance of either route varying in different cultures;
(2) by needle-sticking;
(3) by vertical transmission; and
(4) by blood transfusion.

The last route has been almost completely eliminated in many countries, but may still be an important route in some developing countries.

With most viruses, development of a vaccine involves means to prevent infection by free virus alone. It was realized very early that infection by HIV might involve exposure to both free virus and infected cells. Anderson *et al.* [29] report that HIV-1 has been cultured from different cells in semen, including lymphocytes, granulocytes, monocytes and macrophages. In their study, Anderson *et al.* recovered HIV from the semen of 50% of homosexual HIV-seropositive men and the data supported the conclusion that both free virus and infected cells could transmit the infection. Semen from men with AIDS contained significantly higher levels of total white blood cells, CD4+ lymphocytes and macrophages than semen from seronegative and asymptomatic seropositive men. One AIDS patient had extraordinarily high levels of both free and cell-associated virus in his semen. However, there is great variability in transmission of infection when judged simply by disease symptomatology [22]. Early data suggesting a biologically relevant association between HIV and spermatozoa seem at this stage to be controversial [30, 31].

HIV transmission through semen could be affected by immunosuppressive factors in semen and infection with other viruses. Anti-sperm autoimmunity might induce latently infected cells to express viral antigens or produce infectious virus [29].

Although the rate of recovery of infectious virus from cells is much higher compared to cell-free fluid from serum or plasma [22], presumably both free virus and infected cells in blood can also transmit infection.

(b) *Virus distribution in infected hosts*

The interval between infection and expression of disease varies greatly, possibly from about 3–10 years. There is thus little information about the early distribution of virus in different sites in the body. A variety of cells is now known to be susceptible to infection *in vitro* and virus has been recovered from many different cell types *in vivo* [22]. These include different cells in the brain and a variety of other tissues. Virus has been found in mononuclear phagocytes from blood, brain, lung washings and bone marrow aspirates (e.g. [32]) but reports differ concerning the importance of these cells as a reservoir of infection. McElrath *et al.* [33] consider that monocytes are neither a primary nor an exclusive reservoir of HIV infection, whereas Folks *et al.* [34] have reported that HIV grows in purified progenitor cells of normal human bone marrow. Virus has been isolated from many different body fluids, including urine, saliva, tears and milk. Evidence suggesting that virus may persist in a sanctuary(ies) where it escapes the immune system has been discussed previously [2]; if this effect becomes clearly documented, it strengthens the argument that the time at which a vaccine has maximum opportunity to prevent infection or clear virus should be very shortly after infection occurs.

5.6 THE IMMUNE RESPONSE TO INFECTION BY HIV

Data are now beginning to accumulate on the nature of the immune response to HIV infection and these are briefly outlined now.

5.6.1 Patterns of infection

With acute viral infections in non-immune hosts, viral titres rise to a maximum in target organs within a few days or weeks and then decline and disappear, as the appropriate immune responses are generated. With chronic infections, virus persists at low titres. The situation with HIV is presumed to follow a similar path. That is, viral titres rise to maximum levels some time, at least weeks and possibly months, after initial infection, and then decrease as antibody and effector T cells limit the infection. It was originally thought that infected people made only poor immune responses, but as improved technology for measuring such responses was used it became clear that most people generated strong immune responses for some time after infection so that free virus or antigen may not be found. As the diseases progresses, however, neutralizing antibodies become undetectable, antiviral antibody titres and cytolytic T cell activity decrease and p24 antigenaemia frequently occurs [22].

5.6.2 Detection of antibody

ELISAs (either a sandwich or a competition assay) are now standard procedures for the measurement of antibodies, either to the whole virus or to individual antigens. Western blot analyses are used as a standard to detect false positives by ELISA.

Functional assays, such as neutralization of infectivity, blocking activity, ADCC, or complement-dependent lysis of infected cells are often also used. Of these, particular emphasis is placed on neutralizing antibody as the primary defence mechanism. Although the term neutralization is used to describe an *in vitro* phenomenon, it is widely accepted that this effect occurs *in vivo*. Two types of assays are used to measure this activity — quantal and quantitative [35]. The former includes measuring a reduction in viral antigen production or reverse transcriptase activity in, or immunofluorescence of, infected cells. The endpoint is arbitrarily taken as the last dilution of serum to give a 75–80% reduction. Although our knowledge of the possible different mechanisms involved in viral neutralization is very incomplete (and may vary not only between viruses but also with the Ig isotype), it is not difficult to imagine that *in vitro*, "non-specific" effects such as aggregation of virus by antibody which recognizes "non-neutralizing" epitopes could yield such a loss of activity. Quantitative assays which can accurately measure a 3–4 $\log_{10}$ reduction in plaque numbers or in the formation of syncytia (assuming "one-hit" viral infection kinetics) would be expected to give results which are biologically relevant, as has been seen in many other viral systems. Even with such assays, however, the presence of a very small proportion (<0.01%) of viral mutants would escape detection. Furthermore, unless all viral mutants present at a higher concentration grew well in the cell line used as substrate, they also might not be detected. In fact, although great antigenic variability has clearly been shown to occur in viral samples isolated from an individual over time [36, 37] and most likely in the absence of re-infection, this variability was not seen *in vitro* where a cell line or strain is often used as substrate for virus growth [37]. In contrast, when the envelope regions of six viral clones were separately substituted into a prototype HIV-1 genome, viruses were generated with widely differing capacity to grow in human T cells, cell lines and monocytoid cultures [36].

Both ADCC and complement-dependent lysis of infected cells have been seen when antibody samples from infected people have been assayed *in vitro* [38].

5.6.3 Seroconversion and seroreversion after infection

Shortly after infection, the level of CD4+ cells begins to decline and this fall may continue for some time. It is arrested when neutralizing antibodies appear but their appearance may vary between 4–6 months and 15 months after seroconversion. Generally, no correlation has been observed between the titre of neutralizing antibodies present and progression to disease, but there are some examples where subjects failed to produce any neutralizing antibody and rapidly progressed to AIDS [35]. However, passive immunization with hyperimmune plasma from asymptomatic, healthy patients has now been shown to reverse the progression to disease in some recipients. The transfused patients synthesized antiviral antibody, p24 antigenaemia was cleared and there was a general improvement in their clinical status [39]. This suggests that neutralizing antibody does indeed have an important role in controlling the infection.

One of the initial decisions in the effort to understand the AIDS pandemic was to follow cohorts of people considered to be at great risk of infection. One such group in Baltimore has been followed (with storage and analysis of blood samples) over 2.5 years. Data now shows that 4 members of the cohort, who were originally seropositive, have now become seronegative [40]. Three of these patients have since become polymerase chain reaction (PCR) negative (peripheral blood lymphocytes as substrate; [41]). Not only is this finding encouraging in general, but if virus can be recovered from cell preparations which are PCR+ but seronegative, it will be of great interest to compare the properties of recovered virus compared with both the virus present originally and to the virus present in patients who progress to full-blown AIDS. The nature of the immune response developing in these patients will also be of great interest.

5.6.4 Antibody-mediated immune enhancement

In the presence of antiviral antibody which either fails to neutralize or only poorly neutralizes viral infectivity, agents which replicate productively in cells which possess FcR or CR are likely to show the phenomenon of immune enhancement. This has now been clearly documented with HIV (reviewed in [42]). Compared with the prototype of this phenomenon as seen *in vivo* (dengue virus), where major immunopathological effects occur [43], the observations with HIV *in vitro* are quite minor and probably involve both FcR and CR (e.g. [44–47]). With HIV, the question may not be whether immune enhancement causes a cell to produce more virus, but whether particular cells are more readily infected, thus favouring changes in viral tropism and possibly allowing even a greater diversity of viral variants. Recent *in vitro* experiments [48] show that CD4 immunoadhesins (antibody-like molecules containing the gp120-binding domain of the receptor for HIV linked to the Fc fragment of antibody) block infection by HIV of monocytes with Fc receptors, indicating that the CD4 receptor is the major mechanism for infection of FcR-bearing cells by HIV. Though the effect of immunoadhesins on the pattern of HIV infection has yet to be studied in an *in vivo* system, these findings suggest that immune enhancement may not play a major role in influencing viral replication and distribution *in vivo*.

However, it may be unwise to compare the *in vitro* phenomenon of extent of immune enhancement in the case of an acute infection, like dengue, with an infectious process that may take 10 years to lead to disease. A relatively minor effect seen over a period of days or weeks may greatly influence the course of disease over a decade.

5.6.5   Effector T cell responses

A great amount of work on the cellular immune response to HIV infection has been carried out (summarized in [49, 50]). Work concerning effector T cells capable of controlling viral replication will be discussed here; some aspects have been briefly reviewed elsewhere [2].

Two approaches have been used. The traditional procedure is to measure cytolytic activity of class I MHC-restricted T cells on infected isotope-labelled target cells. A second approach measures the ability of such cells simply to limit or prevent the growth of virus in cells *in vitro*. Several speakers at a recent meeting (MRC AIDS Directed Programme, Cambridge, November 1988) showed that preparations enriched for CD8+ cells from infected people would suppress HIV growth *in vitro* (e.g. [51]).

Cytotoxic T (Tc) cells specific for at least five HIV-specific antigens have been described [2]. A comparison of the reports reporting in detail that the three major proteins, *env*, *pol* and *gag*, are targets for Tc [52–54] indicate that the following points may be general findings:

(1) the PBLs of most asymptomatic HIV-infected people shortly after infection have pronounced Tc activity that is class I MHC-restricted;

(2) this activity is present without restimulation by antigen *in vitro*;

(3) the activity persists for long periods, in some cases for at least two years (C. Flexner, personal communication);

(4) as the symptoms of disease appear and progress, the Tc activity may wane. Some AIDS patients have minimal or no cytotoxic responses [55].

Particular findings include:

(1) peptides have been isolated from *gag* which, in association with HLA-B27, will sensitize target cells [54].

(2) Hoffenbach *et al.* [52] studied the frequency (using limit dilution techniques) in lungs, lymph nodes and blood of activated Tc cells and precursor Tc cells (both were class I MHC-restricted) from asymptomatic and symptomatic AIDS patients. High frequencies of both HIV-specific activated and precursor cells were found in asymptomatic individuals, but the frequencies of both cells decreased as the clinical and immunological status of the patients deteriorated. Surprisingly, PBLs from seronegative individuals yielded high frequencies of HIV-specific Tc cells after *in vitro* stimulation. This has not been observed by others. The effect seems to be limited to the *env* protein and may reflect priming due to other infectious agents or cross-reactivity with normal host components for which there is some evidence (see later). Further to this point, it has also been observed [56] that at least a portion of the cytolytic response against HIV-envelope expressing targets is not major MHC antigen restricted. This particular effect may be due to ADCC.

Siliciano *et al.* [18] made the interesting finding that a subset of CD4+ gp120-specific clones manifest cytolytic activity and lyse uninfected autologous CD4+Ia+ T cells in the presence of gp120 in a process that is strictly dependent upon CD4-mediated uptake of gp120 by T cells. It would be of great interest to know the frequency of primary CD4+ cells showing this activity relative to the corresponding CD8+ cells in infected people.

5.6.6 Suppression of immune responses

Suppressor cell activity in PBLs from patients with AIDS has also been reported (reviewed in [49, 50]), but until recently there has been a lack of detailed information as to whether suppressor activity is generated shortly after infection, leading to a delayed or low antibody response. Using synthetic peptides a region (*env* aa sequence 581–597) within the HIV transmembrane protein, gp41, which specifically inhibits murine and human lymphoproliferation, has now been identified [57]. There is evidence suggesting that, in HIV seropositive individuals, antibody reactivity with this peptide is associated with the absence of disease [58]. Thus, an antibody response against the aa 581–597 region might be capable of abrogating its immunosuppressive effects [57].

5.7 POTENTIAL OBSTACLES TO THE DEVELOPMENT OF AN EFFECTIVE HIV VACCINE

Before discussing possible approaches to vaccine development, this section discusses the potential and perceived major obstacles to the development of an effective vaccine either to prevent or to clear an HIV infection. This is based on the premise that the best chance for a vaccine to be effective is shortly after infection, before the viral load has increased and before the virus has spread through the host and infected a variety of cells.

5.7.1 Antigenic variation

Pronounced antigenic variation — and particularly antigenic drift, where mutations in important B and T cell epitopes arise spontaneously — in the "protective" antigen(s) of an infectious agent has been and remains the major obstacle to the development of vaccines which aim to protect against infection. The classical examples are influenza and rhino viruses. This generally also applies to retroviruses; antibody preparations may neutralize viral infectivity *in vitro*, but the antibody *in vivo* is non-protective [2]. To date, there are no highly successful preventive vaccines against influenza or rhinoviruses.

Despite some findings following immunization with peptides from p17, which will be discussed later, workers in this area attending a recent international meeting agreed that the *env* protein of HIV is the only viral antigen with which neutralizing antibody reacts [35]. For this reason, it is a prime target for inclusion in a vaccine and several candidate vaccines have been prepared which contain this protein, either as a subunit preparation or as a recombinant vaccinia virus. As stated earlier, this protein shows marked antigenic variation. Whereas nucleotide differences between different isolates of HIV differ by at least 13%, i.e. one nucleotide change out of eight [37], the variation in the *env* antigen is thought to be of the order of 26%, i.e. one nucleotide in four. These changes occur in five hypervariable regions of the molecule of which one, 303–337, is stated to be immunodominant, and also in several other regions that show less variability.

Callahan *et al.* [59] have summarized the effects of sequence variability in the T cell epitope, sequence 410–429 of gp120. With some strains, sequence variation altered the interaction of the complex with the TCR. In the case of two highly divergent strains, the variation prevented interaction with DR4 on the antigen-presenting cell.

The following epitopes are thought to be associated with neutralization of HIV-1, as detected with different viral isolates [35]:

(1) RP 135; aa sequence 305–323;
(2) aa sequence 254–274; this epitope is said to be immunosilent in natural HIV infection;
(3) aa sequence 735–752; this epitope is on the intracellular side of the transmembrane domain;
(4) several undefined, presumably conformational epitopes. The *env* protein exists as a trimer, thus enhancing the possibility of important conformational epitopes, as has been shown to be the case with influenza and other viruses (e.g. [10]).

Antibody to region 1 tends to be strain specific, whereas antibody to regions 2 and 3 neutralize several isolates. However, as relatively few monoclonal antibodies that neutralize viral infectivity have been studied, other sites may also prove to be important. It is reported that during the course of infection, neutralizing antibodies are found which are more cross-protective than those found early in the infection [60].

As the *env* protein has a "shroud" of carbohydrate, other regions of the protein, in addition to aa 254–274, may be "immunosilent".

5.7.2   Infection by infected cells

As previously remarked, there is a lack of knowledge of the role of infected cells in transmission of infection. Until more is known about the state of such cells (latent infection, expression of viral antigens, etc.), it is difficult to predict the relative importance of humoral and CMI mechanisms in eliminating the infected cells. Because of the requirement for HLA compatibility, CTL responses would only be effective if the infected cell fused with a host cell.

5.7.3 Immune enhancement: replication in macrophages/monocytes

As the virus replicates in these cells and infected monocytes may be an important mechanism for viral dissemination *in vivo*, mutant virus which escapes neutralization by antibody may be selectively adsorbed to cells expressing CD4, FcR and/or CR, and so gain entry to the cell.

5.7.4 The risk of enhancing infection/immunopathology by vaccination

Several possibilities exist, in addition to that given in Section 5.7.3 above.

(a) *Autoimmune reactions*

The degree of molecular mimicry between the proteins of the host and "foreign" agents is now recognized to be substantially greater than when Burnet first proposed the Clonal Selection Theory. In one study [61], up to 3.5% of monoclonal antibodies prepared against 11 viruses were found to react with normal tissues. It is to be expected that HIV antigens would show amino-acid homologies with sequences in host proteins. This has been demonstrated with the *env* protein. At least three regions of homology have been found — neuroleukin, HLA-DR and interleukin-2. Inclusion of gp160 into a vaccine thus runs a risk of inducing autoimmune reactions. There is at present no way to assess whether autoimmune disease would ensue.

(b) *Antibody-mediated immunopathology*

Gp120 may be shed from the surface of HIV-infected cells and virions [62]. The shed gp120 can bind to CD4+ cells, thus making these cells susceptible to lysis by antiviral antibody and complement.

(c) *Effector T cell-mediated immunopathology*

Activated T cells induce inflammation. There is some evidence that with effector Tc cells, the level of the pathology induced will vary with the extent of viral infection — the fewer the number of infected cells, the less T cell-mediated inflammation [63]. It has been proposed that AIDS is at least partially caused by a T cell-mediated immunopathology in which virus-specific Tc cells destroy virus-infected cells that are involved in immune responses [64]. Siliciano *et al.* [18] have shown that cloned class II MHC-restricted T cells specific for gp120 can lyse CD4 T cells that have been exposed to gp120. On the assumption that gp120 is shed from HIV-infected cells *in vivo*, it was proposed that this novel CD4-dependent autocytolytic mechanism could contribute to the profound depletion of CD4+ cells in AIDS.

If a vaccine that deliberately induced strong Tc cell memory failed to clear virus after infection and the viral load and hence the number of infected cells steadily increased, thus maintaining and perhaps increasing the level of Tc activity, there would be the opportunity for extensive immunopathology.

5.8   APPROACHES TO VACCINE DEVELOPMENT

There are potentially a number of different approaches that can be examined for their feasibility for the development of HIV vaccine(s). They are:

(1) live, attenuated or genetically modified virus, occurring naturally or developed by experimentation;
(2) whole, inactivated virus preparation;
(3) peptide-based preparations which contain either the most suitable B and T cell epitopes, or B cell epitopes conjugated to suitable protein carriers, such as bacterial toxoids;
(4) subunit preparations consisting of one or more of the important antigens of the virus;
(5) live viral or bacterial vectors into which are inserted gene(s) coding for one or more of the HIV antigenic proteins;
(6) anti-idiotope-based preparation, containing one or more anti-idiotypes that are the internal images of important B and possibly T cell epitopes.

In view of the great success of attenuated live viral vaccines to control many viral infections, is it feasible to attempt to generate attenuated live strains of HIV? At present, this is regarded as an unacceptable approach because of the possibility of mutation, and, being a retrovirus, the viral genomic DNA would persist in the host cell genome and presumably be available for recombination with the DNA/cDNA of other retroviral pathogens during possible later infections.

Attempts so far to develop a vaccine based on the anti-idiotype concept have met with very limited success [65] and will not be further discussed here.

5.9 CANDIDATE VACCINES TRIED OR UNDER TRIAL

A number of other approaches have already been tried, are under trial or trials are planned in either model systems or in humans. In addition, some "unusual" approaches have been made.

5.9.1 Animal studies

A number of preparations have been and are being studied in animal models as potential candidate vaccines. In the main experimental animal used, the chimpanzee, it has not been possible so far to generate a protective response by immunization with the *env* antigen. One preparation, gp120 isolated from infected cells, induced antibodies that had weak neutralizing activity [66]. The second preparation was a recombinant vaccinia virus construct containing DNA coding for the gp160 antigen. This preparation induced antibody formation first to the gp41 protein and later to the gp120 protein. No neutralizing antibodies were detected [67]. Specific T helper and Tc cell activity were also generated [68].

In considering these last results, it should be noted that gp160 has been shown to contain an immunodominant epitope recognized by class I MHC-restricted murine Tc cells and that this epitope, aa 308–322, occurs in the highly variable immunodominant region of the molecule [69]. It is also of interest that two peptide sequences, aa 428–443 and aa 112–124 (both in the relatively invariant portion of gp120) were predicted and found to be recognized in mice by class II MHC-restricted T cells. Healthy human volunteers who had been immunized with a recombinant vaccinia virus containing the *env* gene and boosted with a recombinant fragment gave a T cell response to either one or the other of these sequences [70].

Why did the Tc cells generated by the vaccinia construct not protect the chimpanzees from the subsequent challenge? It is possible that though the Tc cells presumably recognized the particular aa sequence 308–322 in the vaccine, mutant viruses may well have arisen after (or been present in) the challenge infection which had different aa sequences and so escaped inactivation by the preformed Tc cells.

Eichberg [71] has reported ongoing immunization experiments in chimpanzees with nine different preparations covering most of the approaches outlined above. None so far has been successful.

More optimism is expressed in a report by Desrosiers *et al.* [72], who multiply immunized rhesus monkeys with whole SIV, inactivated either with formalin or disrupted with detergent and administered with adjuvant. Two of six monkeys immunized with disrupted virus were not infected with challenge virus and three of the other four monkeys, though they became infected, have remained free from disease. All unimmunized monkeys were infected and became diseased. The levels of antibody generated following immunization, and particularly neutralizing antibody, were quite low. The same strain of tissue culture-grown virus was used for both immunization and challenge; though uncloned, other experience suggests [37] that the preparation may not have expressed the same degree of antigen diversity present in the original isolate.

The amino-acid sequence 735–752 of gp41 is conserved on the inside of the viral envelope and is considered to be responsible, at least in part, for the cross-r eutralizing activity observed in people infected for some time (Section 5.7.1). In an ingenious experiment, this sequence has been inserted into the VP1 protein of Sabin type polio virus, replacing a sequential epitope of 12 amino acids which has polio virus neutralizing activity. The chimaeric virus has been found not only to adsorb out much of the cross-neutralizing activity present in sera from infected humans, but also to induce in some hyperimmunized rabbits cross-protective antibodies, albeit to low titre [73]. Protection experiments in chimpanzees are planned.

5.9.2   Human studies

Zagury *et al.* [74, 75] have immunized humans in Africa with a vaccinia virus–HIV gp160 construct followed by a later injection of inactivated, autologous recombinant vaccinia-infected cells. An anamnestic response against HIV was generated that exhibited strong cellular and humoral anti-HIV elements. High levels of antibodies were found to the viral envelope, including broadly reacting neutralizing antibodies. Group-specific CMI and cell-mediated cytotoxicity against infected cells, and hypersensitivity reactions were observed [76]. Though this approach is not feasible on a large scale, the results are promising.

Salk [77, 78] has treated symptomatic individuals with a preparation of inactivated HIV which is deficient in the *env* antigen and has reported on the early results of this treatment [78]. The same preparation has been administered to already infected chimpanzees; virus could not subsequently be recovered from the animals. Re-exposure of these animals to a second virus challenge did not result in superinfection. A third immunized animal became only transiently infected after exposure to virus [79].

Two candidate vaccines are under Phase I trials in human volunteers. One is a gp160 preparation made by recombinant baculovirus-infected insect cells; the second is a recombinant vaccinia virus containing the gene coding for gp160. Volunteers who have either been immunized previously with smallpox vaccine or non-immunized are receiving the recombinant vaccinia virus candidate vaccine. In view of the likelihood that neither vaccine would protect against a challenge infection, it is imperative that the opportunity be taken to assess the safety and biological (including immunological) responses to the candidate vaccines in detail.

Sarin *et al.* [80] found in 1986 that antibody to thymosin $\alpha 1$, a thymic hormone, would neutralize HTLVIII/LAV (HIV). A 44–50% homology was found between the aa sequences 11–28 of thymosin and 92–109 of p17, a conserved sequence of the *gag* protein. It has recently been reported [81] that:

(1) the presence of antibodies to p17 is associated with stabilization and a positive clinical outlook in HIV-infected people;
(2) monoclonal antibodies to this epitope neutralize viral infectivity;
(3) this aa sequence is also a dominant T cell epitope; and
(4) a peptide KLH/conjugate is immunogenic and non-toxic in mice, rabbits, monkeys and chimpanzees.

A Phase I trial with this preparation has now been initiated in a London hospital. The results are awaited with great interest.

5.10 FACTORS INFLUENCING THE DESIGN OF HIV VACCINES

The major factors to be discussed are the humoral immune response and the effector T cell response generated by the vaccine(s), the form of presentation and the need for appropriate animal models.

5.10.1   The humoral response

The generation of neutralizing antibody by a vaccine is traditionally regarded as a crucially important immune response and the earlier discussions in this chapter have not provided any reason to change this view. Assuming a sensitive assay is used (Section 5.6.2), aspects to be considered include:

(1) the efficacy of individual monoclonal antibodies in neutralization of viral infectivity;
(2) the extent of aa sequence variation;
(3) the immunodominance of the region of the antigen;
(4) linear versus discontinuous epitopes; and
(5) cross-protective versus specific epitopes.

A linear, constant region, immunodominant epitope recognized by antibody which, at very low concentrations, effectively neutralizes viral infectivity, is the ideal. The importance of cross-reactive neutralizing antibodies formed during the later stages of asymptomatic infections and recognizing sequences such as 735–752 may soon be determined in the chimaeric polio experiments. Similarly, the clinical trial with the p17 peptide/KLH preparation may yield important results. As of now, however, the dominant epitopes appear to be in the variable regions.

A critical factor not so far evaluated with HIV is the possibility, demonstrated in other viral systems (e.g. [82]), that on a molecular basis, monoclonal antibodies vary considerably in their ability to neutralize viral infectivity. It is important to identify those epitopes which are the targets of monoclonal antibodies which neutralize viral infectivity at the lowest protein concentration. Such a study might identify discontinuous epitopes as being very important, as is the case with many other viruses.

The disulphide-bridged, variable region containing the aa sequence 296–337 is under intensive investigation to assess the extent of variation as seen in a wide variety of isolates. At present, nearly all residues from 305–337 within this sequence seem to be replaceable. Though attempts to predict amino acid replacements in the variable regions of other viruses, such as the haemagglutinin of influenza virus, have been unsuccessful, sequence analysis of this region from a variety of isolates seems now to be yielding a pattern in the amino acid replacements seen. It may be possible to derive from these data and from other data banks of amino acid sequences important in neutralization of viruses [83] an indication as to whether certain amino acid residues are particularly important. If so, a limited number of synthetic sequences may be found which give cross-protective neutralization patterns.

It may also be appropriate to include the immunosuppressive gp41 sequence (Section 5.6.4) in any vaccine in the expectation that pre-existing antibody to this sequence minimizes immunosuppressive effects following infection with virus.

Unusually high titres of antibodies which cooperate with killer cells to destroy virus-infected targets (ADCC) have been found in asymptomatic people [38] and are largely directed against the *env* antigen. A measurable portion of the antibodies is specific for a conserved region of gp120. The extent of the contribution of ADCC to the clearance of virus is not at all clear.

5.10.2 The CMI response

As the *primary* Tc cell responses so far seen in HIV human infections are class I MHC-restricted, a successful vaccine should contain a number of constant region epitopes recognized by such cells. These are most likely to be found in viral antigens other than the gp160, such as the *gag*, *pol* and the regulatory proteins. In view of the likelihood of extensive Ir gene effects in humans, the vaccine should contain as many epitopes as can be shown as a group to give responses in a number of different inbred mouse strains.

5.10.3 Vaccine presentation

To date, infectious agents as immunogens have proved to be the most effective means of generating Tc cell responses and it is encouraging that a recombinant vaccinia preparation has generated such a response in chimpanzees. It seems at present, and hopefully shortly may be confirmed, that a recombinant vaccinia preparation will be an effective way to generate effective Tc cell memory to gp160 in humans. An additional consideration, to be considered at a later stage, is to include genes coding for selected interleukins into the recombinant virus [2].

In contrast, the vaccinia recombinant generated only low levels of total antibody, and no neutralizing antibody responses in the chimpanzee. In view of the need to generate a strong neutralizing antibody response in humans, it may be appropriate to present antigen(s) containing the selected B cell epitopes quite separately in a formulation which induces strong B cell responses. This might be with immunostimulatory complexes (ISCOMS) or with an adjuvant mixture shown to be effective for this purpose.

5.10.4   The need for additional animal models

The main animal model for HIV studies is the chimpanzee but its significance as a disease model remains to be established. Furthermore, these animals are in limited supply, are costly and are an endangered species in their natural habitat [84]. A variety of other animals have been used for related viral systems [85] and this area has recently been reviewed [86]. Studies with SIV in monkeys suggests that this is a useful model for both infection and disease. However, an animal model suitable for HIV studies and available in thousands as distinct from hundreds would enable far more experimentation, with the additional benefit of yielding statistically significant results. The recent development of the SDID-hu mouse, in which mice displaying severe combined immuno-deficiency syndrome are repopulated with human cells, particularly lymphocytes [87, 88], offers the opportunity to follow infection of human cells with HIV *in vivo* at will and in large numbers. Such mice have been infected with HIV-1 [89] and recently were reported to exhibit some of the disease symptoms characteristic of human infections. It may be possible to develop the SCID-hu mouse model to contain a wider variety of human cells, particularly those involved in antigen presentation to T cells.

5.11   CONCLUSIONS

The development of a vaccine to prevent or control HIV-1 infection of humans still faces formidable obstacles. Though there is a steady accumulation of important information about the virus that is highly relevant to vaccine development, there are significant areas of uncertainty and some important aspects, such as infection by infected cells, remain to be studied in greater depth. There are some possibly hopeful signs. From the point of view of humoral immunity, sensitive and quantitative assays for neutralizing antibody estimation are replacing less accurate techniques and important epitopes recognized by neutralizing antibodies are being documented. A determined effort to map all important epitopes on the *env* protein with monoclonal antibodies should show which are the most important to be exploited for vaccine development. Progress is also being made in the mapping of T cell epitopes, particularly for Tc cell recognition, in the other viral antigens.

The availability of the SCID-hu mouse model should complement other animal models and accelerate the assessment of a variety of different approaches to vaccine development.

Perhaps these advances should be regarded with cautious optimism, as presaging a turning point in the struggle to achieve the goal of a safe and effective vaccine.

REFERENCES

1. Ada, G.L. (1989). Vaccines. In *Fundamental Immunology* (W.E. Paul, ed.). Raven Press, New York, p. 985.
2. Ada, G.L. (1989). Prospects for HIV vaccines. *J. AIDS* **1**, 295.
3. Jones, P.D. and Ada, G.L. (1987). Persistence of influenza virus-specific antibody-secreting cells and B cell memory after primary murine influenza virus infection. *Cell. Immunol.* **109**, 53.
4. Gray, D. and Skarvall, H. (1988). B cell memory is short-lived in the absence of antigen. *Nature, Lond.* **336**, 70.
5. Nossal, G.J.V. and Ada, G.L. (1971). *Antigens, Lymphoid Cells and the Immune Response.* Academic Press, New York.
6. Mandel, T.E., Phipps, R.P., Abbot, A. and Tew, J.W. (1980). The follicular dendritic cell: long term antigen retention during immunity. *Immunol. Rev.* **53**, 29.
7. Klaus, G.G.B., Humphrey, J.H., Kunkl, A. and Dongworth, D.W. (1980). The follicular dendritic cell: its role in antigen presentation in the generation of immunological memory. *Immunol. Rev.* **53**, 3.
8. Jerne, N.K. (1984). Idiotypic networks and other preconceived ideas. *Immunol. Rev.* **79**, 5.
9. Van Regenmortel, M.H.V., Altsdchuh. D. and Klug, A. (1986). Influence of local structure on the location of antigenic determinants in tobacco mosaic virus protein. In *Synthetic Peptides as Antigens* (R. Porter and J. Whelan, eds), pp. 76–84. Ciba Foundation Symposium 119. John Wiley and Sons, Chichester.
10. Nestorowicz, A., Laver, W.G. and Jackson, D.C. (1985). Antigenic determinants of influenza virus hemagglutinin. X. A comparison of the physical and antigenic properties of monomeric and trimeric forms. *J. Gen. Virol.* **65**, 1687.
11. Tomasinni, J.E. and Colonno, R.J. (1986). Isolation of a receptor protein involved in attachment of human rhinoviruses. *J. Virol.* **58**, 290.
12. Marwick, C. (1986). Possible defense against the common cold: "Block that receptor site". In *Medical News and Perspectives. J. Am. Med. Soc.* **256**, 967.
13. Whitton, J.L. and Oldstone, M.B.A. (1989). Class I MHC can present an endogenous peptide to cytotoxic lymphocytes. *J. Exp. Med.* **170**, 1033.
14. Gould, K., Cossins, J., Bastin, J., Brownlee, G.G. and Townsend, A. (1989). A 15 amino acid fragment of influenza nucleoprotein synthesized in the cytoplasm is presented to class I restricted cytotoxic T lymphocytes. *J. Exp. Med.* **170**, 1051.
15. Long, E.O. and Jacobsen, S. (1989). Pathways of viral antigen processing and presentation to CTL: defined by the mode of virus entry? *Immunol. Today* **10**, 45.
16. Misko, I.S., Pope, J.H., Hutter, R., Soszynski, T.J. and Kane, R.G. (1984).

HLA-DR-antigen associated restriction of EBV-specific cytotoxic T cell clones. *Int. J. Cancer* **33**, 239.

17. Lukacher, A.E., Morrison, L.A., Braciale, V.L., Malissen, B. and Braciale, T.J. (1985). Expression of specific cytolytic activity by H-2 I region-restricted, influenza-specific T lymphocyte clones. *J. Exp. Med.* **162**, 171.

18. Siliciano, R.F., Lawton, T., Knall, C. *et al.* (1988). Analysis of host–virus interactions in AIDS with anti-gp120 T cell clones: effect of HIV sequence variation and a mechanism for CD4+ depletion. *Cell* **54**, 561.

19. Mullbacher, A. and Ada, G.L. (1987). How do cytotoxic T cells work *in vivo*? *Microb. Pathol.* **3**, 315.

20. Dalgleish, A.G., Beverley, P.C.L., Clapham, P.R., Crawford, D.H., Greaves, M.F. and Weiss, R.A. (1984). The CD4 (T4) antigen is an essential component of the receptor for the AIDS retrovirus. *Nature, Lond.* **312**, 763.

21. Klatzman, D., Champagne, E., Chamerat, S. *et al.* (1984). T-lymphocyte T4 molecule behaves as the receptor for human retrovirus LAV. *Nature, Lond.* **312**, 767.

22. Levy, J. (1989). The human immunodeficiency viruses: detection and pathogenesis. In *AIDS: Pathogenesis and Treatment* (J.A. Levy, ed.), pp. 159–230. Marcel Dekker, New York.

23. Fisher, R.A., Bertonis, J.M., Meier, W. *et al.* (1988). HIV infection is blocked *in vitro* by recombinant soluble CD4. *Nature, Lond.* **331**, 76.

24. Clapham, P.R., Weber, J.N., Whitby, D. *et al.* (1989). Soluble CD4 blocks the infectivity of diverse strains of HIV and SIV for T cells and monocytes but not for brain and muscle cells. *Nature, Lond.* **337**, 368.

25. Watanabe, M., Reimann, K.A., DeLong, P.A., Liu, T., Fisher, R.A. and Letvin, N.L. (1989). Effect of recombinant soluble CD4 in rhesus monkeys infected with simian immunodeficiency virus of macaques. *Nature, Lond.* **337**, 267.

26. Stein, B.S., Gowda, S.D., Lifson, J.D., Penhallow, R.C., Bensch, K.G. and Englemann, E.G. (1987). pH-independent HIV entry into CD4 positive T cells via virus envelope fusion to the plasma membrane. *Cell* **49**, 659.

27. Rabson, A.B. (1989). The molecular biology of HIV infection: clues for possible therapy. In *AIDS: Pathogenesis and Treatment* (J.A. Levy, ed.), p. 231. Marcel Dekker, New York.

28. Haseltine, W.A. and Wong-Staal, F. (1988). The molecular biology of the AIDS virus. *Sci. Am.* **259**(4), 52.

29. Anderson, D.J., Wolff, H., Pudney, J., Zhang, W., Martinez, A. and Mayer, K. (1990). HIV in semen. In *Heterosexual Transmission of AIDS* (N.J. Alexander, H.L. Gabelnick and J.M. Spieler, eds), p. 167.

30. Ashida, E.R. and Scofield, V.L. (1987). Lymphocyte major histocompatibility complex-encoded class II structures may act as sperm receptors. *Proc. Natl Acad. Sci. USA* **84**, 3395.

31. Bagasra, O., Freund, M., Weidmann, J. and Harley, G. (1988). Interaction of human immunodeficiency virus with human sperm *in vitro*. *J. AIDS* **1**, 431.

32. Gartner, S., Markovits, P., Markovitz, D.M., Kaplan, M.H., Gallo, R.C. and Popovic, M. (1986). The role of mononuclear phagocytes in HTLV-III/LAV infection. *Science* **233**, 215.

33. McElrath, M.J., Pruett, J.E. and Cohn, Z.A. (1989). Mononuclear

phagocytes of blood and bone marrow: Comparative roles as viral reservoirs in human immunodeficiency virus type 1 infections. *Proc. Natl Acad. Sci. USA* **86**, 675.

34. Folks, T.M., Kessler, S.W., Orenstein, J.M., Justement, J.S., Jaffe, E.S. and Fauci, S. (1988). Infection and replication of HIV-1 in purified progenitor cells of normal human bone marrow. *Science* **242**, 919.

35. WHO Workshop on the Measurement and Significance of Neutralizing Antibody to HIV and SIV (1990). *Bull. WHO* (accepted for publication).

36. Fisher, A.G., Ensoli, B., Looney, D. *et al.* (1988). Biologically diverse molecular variants within a single HIV-1 isolate. *Nature, Lond.* **334**, 444.

37. Saag, M.S., Hahn, B.H., Gibbons, J. *et al.* (1988). Extensive variation of human immunodeficiency virus type-1 *in vivo*. *Nature, Lond.* **334**, 440.

38. Lyerly, H.K., Reed, D.L., Matthews, T.J. *et al.* (1987). Anti-gp120 antibodies from HIV seropositive individuals mediate broadly reactive anti-HIV ADCC. *AIDS Res. Hum. Retroviruses* **3**, 409.

39. Karpas, A., Hill, F., Youle, M. *et al.* (1988). Effects of passive immunization in patients with the acquired immunodeficiency syndrome-related and acquired immune deficiency syndrome. *Proc. Natl Acad. Sci. USA* **85**.

40. Farzadegan, H., Polis, M.A., Wolinsky, S.M. *et al.* (1988). Loss of human immunodeficiency virus Type 1 (HIV-1) antibodies with evidence of viral infection in asymptomatic homosexual men. *Ann. Intern. Med.* **108**, 785.

41. Farzadegan, H., Wolinsky, S., Sninsky, J. *et al.* (1989). Loss of serologic markers of HIV-1 in asymptomatic HIV-1 infected homosexual men. *Vth International Conference on AIDS*, Montreal, June 1989.

42. Barnes, D. (1988). Another glitch for AIDS vaccines? *Science* **241**, 533.

43. Halstead, S. (1988). Pathogenesis of dengue: challenges to molecular biology. *Science* **239**, 476.

44. Robinson, W.E., Montefiori, D.C. and Mitchell, W.M. (1988). Antibody-dependent enhancement of human immunodeficiency virus type 1 infection. *Lancet* **i**, 790.

45. Gras, G., Strub, T. and Dormont, D. (1988). Antibody-dependent enhancement of HIV infection. *Lancet* **i**, 1285.

46. Takeda, A., Tuazon, C.U. and Ennis, F.A. (1988). Antibody-enhanced infection by HIV-1 via Fc receptor-mediated entry. *Science* **242**, 580.

47. Homsy, J., Tateno, M. and Levy, J.A. (1988). Antibody-dependent enhancement of HIV infection. *Lancet* **i**, 1285.

48. Capon, D.J., Chamow, S.M., Mordenti, J. *et al.* (1989). Designing CD4 immunoadhesins for AIDS therapy. *Nature, Lond.* **337**, 525.

49. Krowka, J.F., Moody, D.J. and Stites, D.P. (1989). Immunological effects of HIV infection. In *AIDS: Pathogenesis and Treatment* (J.A. Levy, ed.), p. 257. Marcel Dekker, New York.

50. Sattentau, Q.J. (1990). Molecular interactions between CD4 and the HIV envelope glycoproteins. In *AIDS and the New Viruses* (G. Dalgleish and R. Weiss, eds), pp. 41–53. Academic Press, London.

51. Walker, C.M., Moody, D.J., Stites, D.P. and Levy, J.A. (1986). CD8 lymphocytes can control HIV infection *in vitro* by suppressing virus replication. *Science* **234**, 1563.

52. Hoffenbach, A., Langlade-Demoyen, P., Dadaglio, G. *et al.* (1989). Unusually high frequencies of HIV-specific cytotoxic T lymphocytes in humans. *J. Immunol.* **142**, 452.

53. Walker, B.D., Flexner, C., Paradis, T.J. *et al.* (1988). HIV-1 reverse transcriptase is a target for cytotoxic T lymphocytes in infected individuals. *Science* **240**, 64.
54. Nixon, D.F., Townsend, A.R.M., Elvin, J.G., Rizza, C.R., Gallwey, J. and McMichael, A.J. (1988). HIV-1 gag-specific cytotoxic T lymphocytes defined with recombinant vaccinia virus and synthetic peptides. *Nature, Lond.* **336**, 484.
55. Koenig, S. (1989). Cytotoxic T-cell responses to the virus HIV. p. 377–8. In (A.S. Fauci, moderator) Development and evaluation of a vaccine for human immunodeficiency virus infection. *Ann. Intern. Med.* **110**, 373.
56. Koenig, S., Earl, P., Powell, D. *et al.* (1988). Group specific, major histocompatibility complex class I restricted cytotoxic responses to human immunodeficiency virus-1 envelope proteins by cloned peripheral blood T cells from an HIV-infected individual. *Proc. Natl Acad. Sci. USA* **85**, 8638.
57. Ruegg, C.L., Monell, C.R. and Strand, M. (1989). Inhibition of lympho-proliferation by a synthetic peptide with sequence identity to gp41 of human immunodeficiency virus type 1. *J. Virol.* **63**, 3257.
58. Klasse, P.J., Pipkorn, R. and Blomberg, J. (1988). Presence of antibodies to a putatively immunosuppressive part of human immunodeficiency virus (HIV) envelope glycoprotein gp41 is strongly associated with health among HIV-positive subjects. *Proc. Natl Acad. Sci. USA* **85**, 5225.
59. Callahan, K.M., Fort, M., Obah, E.A., Reinherz, E.L. and Siliciano, R.F. (1990). Genetic variability in HIV-1 affects interactions with HLA molecules and T cell receptors. *J. Immunol.* **144**, 3341.
60. Weiss, R.A., Clapham, P.R., Weber, J.N. *et al.* (1986). Variable and conserved neutralization antigens of human immunodeficiency virus. *Nature, Lond.* **324**, 572.
61. Srinivasappa, J., Prabhakar, B.S., Essani, K. *et al.* (1986). Molecular mimicry: frequency of reactivity of monoclonal antiviral antibodies with normal tissues. *J. Virol.* **57**, 397.
62. Schneider, I., Kaaden, O., Copeland, T.D., Oroslan, S. and Hunsmann, G. (1986). Shedding and interspecies type sero-reactivity of the envelope glycopeptide gp120 of the human immunodeficiency virus. *J. Gen. Virol.* **67**, 2533.
63. Mak, N.K., Sweet, C., Ada, G.L. and Tannock, G.A. (1983). The sensitization of mice with a wild-type and cold-adapted variant of influenza virus. II. Secondary cytotoxic T cell responses. *Immunology* **51**, 407.
64. Zinkernagel, R.M. (1989). Virus-triggered AIDS: a T-cell-mediated immuno-pathology? *Immunol. Today* **9**, 370.
65. Kennedy, R.C. (1989). Strategies to develop idiotype-based vaccines against human immunodeficiency virus (Abstract). *1989 Annual Meeting*, Laboratory of Tumour Cell Biology, National Cancer Institute, Bethesda, MD.
66. Arthur, L.O., Pyle, S.W., Nara, P.L. *et al.* (1987). Serological responses in chimpanzees inoculated with human immunodeficiency virus glycoprotein (gp120) subunit vaccine. *Proc. Natl Acad. Sci. USA* **84**, 8583.
67. Hu, S.L., Fultz, P.N., McClure, H.M. *et al.* (1987). Effect of immunization with a vaccinia-HIV *env* recombinant on HIV infection of chimpanzees. *Nature, Lond.* **328**, 721.
68. Zarling, J.M., Eichberg, J.W., Moran, P.A., McClure, J., Srider, P. and Hu, S.L. (1987). Proliferative and cytotoxic T-cells to AIDS virus glyco-

proteins in chimpanzees immunized with a recombinant vaccinia virus expressing AIDS virus envelope glycoproteins. *J. Immunol.* **139**, 988.

69. Takahashi, H., Cohen, J., Hosmalin, A. *et al.* (1988). An immunodominant epitope of the human immunodeficiency virus envelope glycoprotein gp160 recognized by class 1 major histocompatibility complex molecule restricted murine cytotoxic T lymphocytes. *Proc. Natl Acad. Sci. USA* **85**, 3105.

70. Berzofsky, J.A., Benussan, A., Cease, K.B. *et al.* (1988). Antigenic peptides recognized by T lymphocytes from AIDS viral envelope-immune humans. *Nature, Lond.* **334**, 706.

71. Eichberg, J.W. (1989). Active and passive immunization against HIV in chimpanzees (Abstract). *1989 Annual Meeting*, Laboratory of Tumour Biology, National Cancer Institute, Bethesda, MD.

72. Desrosiers, R.C., Wyand, M.S., Kodama, T. *et al.* (1989). Vaccine protection against simian immunodeficiency virus infection. *Proc. Natl Acad. Sci. USA* **86**, 6353.

73. Evans, D.J., McKeating, J., Meredith, J.M. *et al.* (1989). An engineered poliovirus chimera elicits broadly reactive HIV-1 neutralizing antibodies. *Nature, Lond.* **339**, 385.

74. Zagury, D., Leonard, R., Fouchard, M. *et al.* (1987). Immunization against AIDS in humans. *Nature, Lond.* **326**, 249.

75. Zagury, D., Bernard, J., Chenier, R. *et al.* (1988). A group-specific anamnestic reaction against HIV-1 induced by a candidate vaccine against AIDS. *Nature, Lond.* **332**, 728.

76. Gallo, R.C., Bolognesi, D.P. and Nerurkar, L.S. (1989). The immune response to infection with HIV. In (A.S. Fauci, moderator) Development and evaluation of a vaccine for human immunodeficiency virus infection. *Ann. Intern. Med.* **110**, 373.

77. Salk, J. (1987). Prospects for the control of AIDS by immunizing seropositive individuals. *Nature, Lond.* **327**, 473.

78. Salk, J. (1989). The whole virus approach to immunization. In (A.S. Fauci, moderator) Development and evaluation of a vaccine for human immunodeficiency virus infection. *Ann. Intern. Med.* **110**, 378.

79. Research News (1989). New hope on the AIDS vaccine front. *Science* **244**, 1254.

80. Sarin, P.S., Sun, D.K., Thornton, A.H., Naylor, P.H. and Goldstein, A.L. (1986). Neutralization of HTLVIII.LAV replication by antiserum to thymosin 1. *Science* **232**, 1135.

81. Goldstein, A.L., Naylor, P.H., Gibbs, C.J. and Sarin, P.S. (1989). Progress in the development of HGP-30: an HIV-p17 based vaccine (Abstract). *1989 Annual Meeting*, Laboratory of Tumour Cell Biology, National Cancer Institute, Bethesda, MD.

82. Acharya, R., Fry, E., Stuart, D., Fox, G., Rowlands, D. and Brown, F. (1989). The three dimensional structure of foot-and-mouth disease virus at 2.9 Å resolution. *Nature, Lond.* **337**, 709.

83. Geyson, H.M., Rodda, S.J. and Mason, T.J. (1986). The delineation of peptides able to mimic assembled epitopes. In *Synthetic Peptides as Antigens* (R. Porter and J. Whelan, eds), p. 130. John Wiley and Sons, New York.

84. WHO Consultation on the Need for International Testing of HIV Vaccines (1989). WHO, Geneva.

85. Kurth, R., Kraus, G., Werner, G. *et al.* (1989). AIDS: Animal retrovirus models and vaccines. *J. AIDS* **1**, 284.
86. Purcell, R.H. (1989). Animal models for the development of a vaccine for the acquired immunodeficiency syndrome. In (A.S. Fauci, moderator) Development and evaluation of a vaccine for human immunodeficiency virus infection. *Ann. Intern. Med.* **110**, 373.
87. McCune, J.M., Namikawa, R., Kaneshima, H. *et al.* (1988). The SCID-hu mouse: murine model for the analysis of human hematolymphoid differentiation and function. *Science* **241**, 1632.
88. Mosier, D.E., Gulizia, R., Baird, S. and Wilson, D. (1988). Transfer of a functional human immune system to mice with severe combined immunodeficiency. *Nature, Lond.* **335**, 256.
89. Namikawa, R., Kaneshima, M., Lieberman, M., Weissman, I.L. and McCune, J.M. (1988). Infection of SCID-hu mice by HIV-1. *Science* **242**, 1684.

6 | The Pathogenesis of HIV-induced Disease

ANGUS G. DALGLEISH, FABRIZIO MANCA AND
JOHN A. HABESHAW

*Retroviral Research Group, Clinical Research Centre,
Watford Road, Harrow HA1 3UJ, UK*

6.1 INTRODUCTION

In spite of the detailed understanding of the cell and molecular biology of human immunodeficiency virus (HIV) reviewed in previous chapters, we still do not understand the reasons why HIV takes a mean of 8–10 years to cause disease in those infected. Most viruses cause an acute infection from which the host usually recovers; occasionally the infection causes the host to die. Only rarely do long-term sequelae follow. For example, the human retrovirus HTLV-1 is associated with adult T cell leukaemia and tropical spastic paraparesis in only about 1% of those infected, as reviewed by Schultz and Weber in Chapter 7. The time period between infection and disease is estimated to be of the order of several decades, with the exception of a few cases where the virus has been contracted by blood transfusion, when the disease occurs within a few years. Another example is the Epstein Barr virus (EBV); most people exposed in early life develop no disease, whereas delay till adolescence or later often results in glandular fever, in most cases without further sequelae developing. However, in some parts of the world EBV is clearly associated with the development of the malignancies Burkitt's lymphoma and nasopharyngeal carcinoma. Co-factors are probably involved as the tumours have defined geographical distributions and ethnic bias. Even so, clinical disease is still a rare consequence of EBV infection. Herpes simplex, cytomegalo-virus and hepatitis B virus also cause persistent infection, the last clearly being associated with hepatoma in a minority of people infected.

In Chapter 2, Haseltine reviews the current state of our understanding of the molecular biology of HIV and suggests that progressive disease is a consequence of the gradual rise in the virus replication rate after a prolonged period of attenuated replication. A dynamic model is suggested whereby known properties of HIV may be accounted for by the slow and inexorable switch from controlled to prolific replication. Most HIV infections of resting CD4 cells are latent. However, subsequent

AIDS AND THE NEW VIRUSES
ISBN 0–12–200740–9

activation of the cell leads to virus replication and dissemination. The gradual selection of virus variants which grow in specific cell lines is also thought to be an important factor in the pathogenesis of disease.

Virus isolation from patients can be achieved with varying degrees of difficulty, depending on the patient. It is usually easier to isolate HIV from patients with AIDS than from those who remain asymptomatic [1, 2]. Following isolation, viruses have been noted to be either fast replicators and relatively cytopathic or slow replicators with little cytopathogenicity [3]. A change over time with viruses changing from "slow" to "fast" as disease progresses has also been reported [4]. The initial and changing cellular tropism of the virus is thought to have major implications for the pathogenesis of disease. Some isolates are more monocytotropic than lymphocytotropic, and vice versa [5]. Isolates with different tropisms have been isolated from different sites in the same individual [6]. Tissue tropisms have been reported to be associated with specific amino acid changes in the envelope [7], as well as different nuclear and transcriptional binding characteristics [8]. As more than one factor is involved, it is likely that the tropism *in vivo* is relative rather than absolute.

6.2   *IN VIVO* MUTATION OR QUASI-SPECIES?

Do these different isolates evolve in the host, or does the host become infected with a variety of different isolates that are then subjected to different selection pressures? In the first instance it is assumed that an infecting isolate would be of the slow variety (or else the "fast" isolates are "dealt with" by the immune system and the "slow" isolates survive) and the rate of replication adequately controlled by the immune response until it escapes neutralization and other controls by developing mutations in the highly variable regions of the envelope [9]. Thus a fast cytopathic isolate would become dominant early in the disease. If this model was the only explanation for the long latency, then the virus could be expected to increase in virulence. In other words, the more cytopathic isolates would become dominant, in populations as well as in individuals, who would have a very short latency period from infection to disease. Therefore, more aggressive isolates might be expected to be isolated from recently infected individuals.

The concept that the host is infected with a variety of different related yet distinct HIV viral genomes known as quasi-species has been suggested by Wain-Hobson and is based on an original observation with vesicular stomatitis viruses by Holland [10, 11]. The main evidence comes from restriction mapping of molecularly cloned proviruses [12]. Dominant isolates with many minor isolates can be isolated from many different anatomical sites, and these dominant isolates may change over several months *in vivo* [13], although a "founder" effect with a few clones that undergo divergence could still apply.

The HIV genome variations are equally complex in both asymptomatic and AIDS patients, although the ability of the virus to grow in culture improves as the CD4 count declines *in vivo* [14]. However, there are differences between virus populations *in vivo* and *in vitro* which may be due to one or all of the following:

(1) the fastest growing genome has been selected;
(2) IL-2 culture selects against monocytotropic isolates;
(3) IL-2 expands CD8 cells which may kill major yet spare minor forms.

A longitudinal study by Meyerhans *et al.* showed that frequencies of the major forms fluctuated in a way that was independent of the CD4 count [14]. This could be due to a rapid turnover of latently infected cells, either by activation followed by immune destruction or simply destruction as the T cells are regenerated, i.e. killing T cell clones versus HIV clones. An interesting feature of these population studies is the high number of defective viruses that are present [14]. This has two major implications for the pathogenesis of disease. First, many of the defects have been found in the *tat* region (probably due to the fact that it has been analysed so extensively). Recently defective *tat* mutants have been shown to inhibit wild-type virus replication [15]. Second, defective viruses, along with helper viruses, have been shown to cause immunosuppression in both feline and murine leukaemia virus-infected animals [16]. Far from explaining the enigmas of HIV-induced disease, this additional information indicates how complex the pathogenesis of persistent viral infections can be.

6.3 NON-MOLECULAR BASED EXPLANATIONS OF PATHOGENESIS

In Chapter 3, Sattentau discusses the relevance of the gp120–CD4 interaction in HIV infection and he reviews some of the mechanisms whereby CD4 function maybe impaired indirectly. Inhibition of CD4 function by virus, or more specifically the envelope gp120, is attractive as functional impairment prior to detectable falls in CD4 levels can be detected in infected individuals [17]. Moreover, indirect mechanisms of destruction could explain why CD4 levels fall even when few cells can be shown to be even latently infected with the virus [18].

These and other indirect mechanisms of immune destruction will be reviewed briefly:

(1) Uninfected CD4+ cells may be killed by fusing with infected cells [19].

(2) Antigen-presenting cells such as those of the monocyte–macrophage lineage may be infected by HIV [19]. In the absence of cytopathic killing, latently infected cells may be unable to present antigen efficiently. Furthermore, antigen presentation may be accompanied by the transference of HIV genome to a newly activated T cell. Persistent infection interfering with cellular functions that occur after the cell has differentiated has been well described for the lymphocytic choriomeningitis virus, and thus may also be relevant to HIV [20].

(3) The presence of gp120 adhering to CD4 cells may allow these cells to be subjected to cytotoxic attack, either directly [21] or mediated by antibodies against the envelope (ADCC) [22]. Gp120 may interfere with normal CD4 function, either due to down-regulation of the CD4 molecule [19] or by directly interfering with its normal function — antigen recognition in the context of class II MHC antigens [23]. Gp120 may have direct immunosuppressive characteristics similar to those described for the p15E protein of other retroviruses [24]. Interestingly in HIV, gp41, not gp120, is the homologue of p15E.

(4) HIV infection is associated with the induction of autoantibodies which may lead to the destruction of CD4 cells as well as others bearing cross-reactive epitopes [25]. This may explain the thrombocytopenia seen in AIDS.

(5) Indirect mechanisms such as suppression by cytokine induction, cell destruction by cytokines, presence of lymphotoxic serum factors and antibody enhancement of virus infection may all contribute to CD4 cell depletion [26–28].

Some of these mechanisms will now be considered in more detail.

HIV induces fusion of CD4+ cells in culture, leading to the formation of giant multi-nucleated cells known as syncytia [19]. A single virus-producing cell can cause many uninfected CD4+ cells to fuse and die. The cloned envelope gene alone expressed in a suitable cell line will cause the fusion of numerous other CD4+ cells [29]. It should be noted that some cells will undergo cytolysis without involving other cells following infection with HIV, and that cells that survive either process may become chronically infected [30].

It is not known how important fusion-related cell killing is *in vivo*; giant cells are uncommon *in vivo*, although they have been seen in lymph nodes and the brain post-mortem and more frequently in SIV-infected monkeys. Syncytial formation clearly involves CD4 and the HIV envelope, as only the latter is required to induce syncytia, and antibodies against CD4 will inhibit syncytial formation [19]. However, fusion *per se* is an event occurring after CD4–gp120 binding; it can be inhibited by antibodies against the HIV envelope epitopes that do not involve the CD4 binding site. Fusion probably involves at least two sites on gp120 and at least one site on gp41 [31, 32], which may bind to gp120 as well as to other cellular ligands in the process of fusion and penetration. As discussed in Chapter 3, the CD4 molecule may be involved in fusion as well as in gp120 binding. Other molecules are probably involved, as mouse cells expressing CD4 bind but do not become infected with HIV [33]. A possible contender molecule is the lymphocyte functional activation molecule (LFA-1), which appears to be involved in some HIV fusion events, although it is not essential, being absent on HeLa cells expressing CD4, which readily fuse and become infectable with HIV [34, 33]. It may therefore merely indicate that cells must agglutinate before they are close enough to fuse. Understanding the subtle differences between infection with and without obvious fusion may be important to the understanding of the pathogenesis of HIV. However, most retroviruses cause similar fusion of receptor-bearing cells and they have markedly different pathogeneses.

6.4 THE gp120–CD4 INTERACTION

The gp120–CD4 interaction may well affect the function of the CD4 molecule without infecting and killing the cell. First, the CD4 molecule has a pivotal role in immune regulation, and second, most immune responses are impaired in HIV infection, many before the CD4 T cell count has fallen [35]. Whereas the two are undoubtedly linked, the key question is whether or not direct killing of CD4 cells is required to produce a significant immunodeficiency. The role of antigen-presenting cells has already been mentioned; even though they may not necessarily be killed upon infection they may pass HIV to a T cell during the act of antigen presentation, which by definition activates the T cell, a known prerequisite for HIV infection. CD4 function may be reduced by the simple act of down-regulation following infection, thus reducing the number of CD4 molecules for normal immunoregulatory function [19, 23, 35].

Gp120 binds to the CD4 molecule with a higher affinity (10^{-9}M) than does the natural ligand of CD4 — the MHC class II molecule — which binds with an affinity less than 10^{-7}M [36].

The envelope of HIV is readily shed from the virus, although some isolates shed larger amounts of gp120 than others [37]. Free soluble gp120 in the serum has not been reported, which should not be surprising given the large numbers of CD4 molecules available *in vivo* and the high affinity of attraction. Interference of class II MHC–CD4 interactions by gp120 could therefore lead to interference of T cell recognition. Interference with the physiological CD4–MHC class II interaction is enough to produce unresponsiveness of specific T cell lines to foreign antigen presented in association with MHC class II [38]. Gp120 will specifically inhibit CD4-transfected MHC class II-restricted T cell hybridoma cells to antigen, but does not inhibit proliferative responses mediated through CD2 [39].

The inhibitory effect of gp120 on antigen-driven responses has been reported in a number of systems [40–42]. We have recently been able to show that antigen-specific induced activation can be blocked by soluble gp120 and that this inhibition can be prevented by soluble CD4 [43]. Using two specific T cell lines (Tetanus toxoid and PPD), we presented antigen in the presence and absence of HIV gp120 or whole virus, before expanding these lines in IL-2 for several days prior to re-presenting antigen in the absence of HIV. Only those cells which first saw antigen in the absence of HIV or gp120 responded when presented with the specific antigen. By using two specific cell lines we were able to demonstrate how specific the responses inhibited by HIV were, in marked contrast to some earlier reports [44]. Furthermore, we could show that this effect is entirely due to gp120 interacting with the CD4 of the T cell-specific lines and that this response is not affected when HIV or gp120 is pre-incubated on the antigen-presenting cell, prior to antigen presentation.

Lymphocytes are rendered unresponsive to antigen by gp120 alone in the absence of toxicity, making mechanisms via CD4 a likely mode of action [43]. Both positive and negative signalling can be mediated by different regions of the CD4 molecule [23]. Further experiments should help define the model most relevant to gp120.

The failure of an antigen-specific T cell to respond to antigen in the presence of gp120 indicates that CD4, CD3, the T cell receptor (TCR) and MHC class II are all involved in the inhibition by gp120 [45]. During the act of antigen presentation, antigen is presented as a peptide by the MHC class II molecules to the T cell receptor [46]. It is likely that the CD4–MHC class II interaction exists to stabilize or enhance this association [47]. There is certainly an association between CD4 and CD3, as during antigen presentation CD4 and CD3 co-modulate [48]. In contrast, CD2 is not involved and CD2 pathways are not inhibited by HIV or gp120 [49]. The association of the cellular ligands during antigen presentation is shown in Fig. 6.1.

The implications of such specific impairment are as follows: first, recall responses are more likely to be effected than impairment of new antigen presentation; and second, if antigen-specific presentation is inhibited by gp120, then it is possible that gp120 may be able to distort the stereochemistry of the CD3, CD4 class II interaction. The clinical picture of indigenous infections such as candida albicans and pneumocystis pneumonia is in keeping with the impaired recall response. It is of interest that AIDS patients tend to die of diseases endemic in their early environment, hence tuberculosis is common in African AIDS and fungal infections are common in AIDS patients who were born in the American mid-west [50].

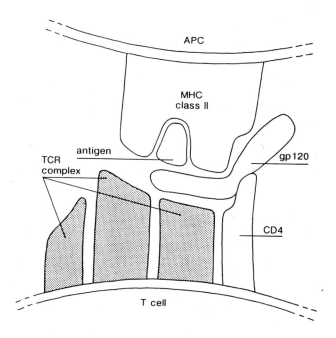

Fig. 6.1 Model for gp120-mediated inhibition of T cell response. Antigen is presented as peptide by MHC class II molecule of APC to the TCR–CD4 complex on T cell. Close association is perturbed by high-affinity binding of gp120 to CD4, which may interfere with TCR recognition of MHC class II plus antigen. TCR = T cell receptor.

With regard to the distorted interpretation of self-MHC antigens, it has been known for some time that cytotoxic responses specific for self+ influenza are markedly impaired early in an infection, in contrast to the well-preserved responses to allo+ influenza, a finding which could be expected when antigen presentation to CD3–TCR is impaired due to distorted recognition of self-MHC class II antigens [51].

6.5   IS AIDS A GRAFT VERSUS HOST (GVH) DISEASE?

The similarities between AIDS and GVH disease were noted by Shearer and colleagues before HIV had been isolated [52]. The clinical features of chronic GVH include skin involvement, diarrhoea, lymphoid depletion, opportunistic infections and lymphomas, all of which are associated with HIV infection. CD4 depletion would result from cytotoxic responses which lyse cells in the presence of gp120.

Such a scenario has already been demonstrated by Siliciano and colleagues, who showed that CD4+ gp120-specific clones could lyse autologous CD4 and HLA DR+ T cells in the presence of gp120, a process dependent on the CD4-mediated uptake of gp120 by T cells [21]. This mechanism of CD4 depletion is similar to syngeneic GVH disease, in which there is isogenotypic identity between the donor and recipient and a GVH reaction occurs against non-HLA antigens such as those of viral or bacterial origin. Apart from the killing of uninfected cells, CD4 levels may be depleted by failure to repopulate due to altered self-recognition by CD4 selection processes in the thymus that may be either autoaggressive or due to a maturation defect (for a further review see [53]).

6.6   OTHER MECHANISMS OF HIV PATHOGENESIS

Although inhibition of antigen-specific responses or distorted recognition of self can be interpreted to offer explanations for some of the more puzzling aspects of HIV pathogenesis, they clearly do not account for all the clinical features seen in HIV infection. Whereas uncontrolled replication of HIV is likely to cause cytopathic events in AIDS patients, the mechanisms of dementia, cachexia and many other features seen in HIV disease probably require more subtle explanations than those provided by direct cytopathic or indirect immunosuppressive mechanisms. Cachexia is commonly seen in cancer patients; the product associated with the onset of cachexia, cachexin, is very similar to tumour necrosis factor (TNF). Recent studies [54–57] have shown that TNF (along with γ-interferon (γ-IFN) can induce HIV-1 production in tumour cell lines and peripheral blood mononuclear cells. However, HIV-1 can also induce cytokine induction including TNF and γ-IFN secretion [57].

The ability of cytokines to influence HIV replication and HIV to affect cytokine production open up many other possibilities to describe the pathogenesis of HIV infection. The functions of cytokines are diverse and heavily dependent on many other factors within their ambit of operation. In this regard it is important to appreciate that cytokines have very narrow ranges of action (i.e. <2 mm), have very short half-lives, and usually require specific receptors on their host cells' surface [58]. Obviously enhanced levels of TNF secretion could be involved in the development of the cachexia most commonly associated with gastro-enteropathic AIDS, or "slim" disease as it is known in some parts of Africa.

Local induction of cytokines by infected macrophages or lymphocytes may also be in part responsible for the neuro-degenerative changes seen in HIV infection. Indeed, it is not known whether certain cytokine combinations could enhance infectibility of CD4− cells. The complexity of potential cytokine interactions in HIV-infected patients can be judged from the fact that although TNF can enhance HIV replication in cell lines, in combination with γ-IFN it can lyse HIV-infected tumour cells [59]!

Furthermore, cytokines may play an important role in the cytopathic effects of HIV (antibodies against TNF and γ-IFN can inhibit syncytial formation [57]), as well as being involved in antigen-specific activational mechanisms discussed earlier in this chapter. Antigen-activated T cells release lymphokines such as granulocyte–monocyte colony-stimulating factor that can enhance replication in antigen-presenting cells that carry the virus [60–62]. Cytokine induction by HIV has even been proposed as a mechanism for the induction of Kaposi's sarcoma (KS) and increased cytokine production with autocrine and paracrine growth effects have been reported from cells derived from AIDS-associated KS [63].

6.7   IMPLICATIONS FOR HIV TREATMENT AND VACCINE DEVELOPMENT

A consequence of GVH disease is a restricted immune response, and there are several reports of restricted immune responses in HIV infection [64–67]. In particular, the response to the envelope is considerably more restricted than to other HIV antigens such as *gag*. This may be in part due to the fact that the envelope interacts with the CD4 antigen and could, therefore, prevent accurate recognition of itself. This may explain why cytotoxic responses to the T cell epitopes are much weaker than expected [67].

In addition, there are regions of considerable homology between gp160 and self such as MHC class II and IL-2. Indeed, one of the regions of gp120 homologous to class II may well be important in the distorted recognition of self MHC class by CD4 and CD3, i.e. it sees self + gp120 as distorted self MHC rather than self + gp120, which could set in motion those network changes which eventually lead to a chronic GVH disease.

Therapeutically it will be important to reduce the amount of free envelope protein, both by inhibiting virus replication directly (see Chapter 4) as well as preventing any further contact with gp120. This may be possible if soluble CD4 can be maintained at constant serum levels. Apart from its ability to attach to gp120 with an affinity similar to natural CD4, it is also able to neutralize directly a broad range of isolates [68]. A constant level of CD4 might well be able to prevent further antigen unresponsiveness.

Vaccination against HIV should aim at preventing activation of T cell subsets involved in the autosuppressive circuits through which GVH is thought to be mediated, by inducing blocking responses. This has recently been achieved in a mouse GVH model [69]. In more immediate terms, inducing a response against the CD4 binding site may have a similar effect [70].

A further consequence of the gp120–CD4 interactions on the pathogenesis of HIV infection is that the restricted envelope responses will favour non-essential epitopes and that the binding and fusion sites may not be seen by the natural immune response, a scenario we know to be the case *in vivo*. It may be necessary, therefore, to interfere with the gp120–CD4 interaction before immunizing with important protective epitopes whenever they are more clearly defined. Without such an approach, protective vaccines against HIV in chimpanzees (who do not get HIV-related disease) and against the SIV in monkey models may not be relevant to HIV infection in man, due to the fact that the pathogenesis of disease differs subtly in each case. It will be important to bear this in mind as the vaccine approaches reviewed here in Chapter 5 by Ada are gradually tried out in the clinical situation.

REFERENCES

1. Lange, J.M.A., Paul, D.A., De Wolf, F., Coutinho, R.A. and Goudsmidt, J. (1987). Viral gene expression, antibody production and immune complex formation in HIV infection. *AIDS* **1**, 15–20.
2. Farthing, C., Dalgleish, A.G., Clark, A., McClure, M., Chanas, A. and Gazzard, B.G. (1987). Foscarnet (Phosphonformate): a pilot study in AIDS and AIDS related complex. *AIDS* **1**, 21–26.
3. Asjo, B., Morfeldt, L., Manson, L. *et al.* (1986). Replicative capacity of HIV for patients with varying severity of HIV infection. *Lancet* **ii**, 660–662.
4. Cheng-Mayer, C., Seto, D., Talano, M. and Levy, J.A. (1988). Biologic features of HIV-1 that correlate with virulence in the host. *Science* **40**, 80–82.
5. Popovic, M. and Gartner, S. (1987). Isolation of HIV-1 from monocytes but not from T-lymphocytes. *Lancet* **ii**, 916.
6. Chiodi, F., Valentin, A., Keys, B. *et al.* (1990). Biological characteristics of pairs HIV-1 isolates from blood and CSF. *Virology* (in press).
7. Cordonnier, A., Montangnieu, L. and Ememan, M. (1989). Single amino acid changes in the HIV envelope affect viral tropism and receptor binding. *Nature, Lond.* **340**, 571–574.
8. O'Brien, W.A., Koyanagi, Y. and Chen, I.S.Y. (1989). Mechanism of HIV-1 infection of mononuclear phagocytes. *Vth International Conference on AIDS*, Montreal, June 1989 (Abstract T.C.O. 16).
9. Weiss, R.A., Clapham, P.R., Weber, J.N., Dalgleish, A.G., Laskey, L.A. and Berman, P. (1986). Variable and conserved neutralisation antigens of HIV. *Nature, Lond.* **324**, 572–575.
10. Steinhauer, D.A. and Holland, J.J. (1986). Rapid evaluation of RNA viruses. *Ann. Rev. Microbiol.* **41**, 409–433.
11. Wain-Hobson, S. (1989). HIV genome variability *in vitro*. *AIDS* **3** (Suppl. 1), 513–518.
12. Saag, M.S., Halin, B.H., Gibbons, J. *et al.* (1988). Extensive variation of HIV-1 *in vivo*. *Nature, Lond.* **334**, 440–444.
13. Goodenow, M., Hinet, T., Savrin, W., Kurok, S., Sninsky, J.J. and Wain-Hobson, S. (1989). HIV-1 isolates one rapidly evolving quasi-species. *J. AIDS* **2**, 344–352.
14. Meyerhans, A., Cheynier, R., Albert, J. *et al.* (1989). Temporal fluctuations in HIV quasi-species *in vivo* are not reflected by sequential HIV isolation. *Cell* **58**, 901–910.
15. Green, M., Ishino, M. and Lowerstein, P.M. (1989). Mutational analysis of HIV-1 *tat* minimal domain peptides; identification of *trans* dominant mutants that suppress HIV-LTR clinical gene expression. *Cell* **58**, 205–214.
16. Huang, M., Simard, C. and Jolicoeur (1989). Immunodeficiency and clonal growth of target cells induced by helper free defective retrovirus. *Science* **246**, 1614–1618.
17. Fauci, A.S. (1989). The pathogenesis of AIDS. *Science* **239**, 617–622.
18. Harper, M.E., Marselle, L.M., Gallo, R.C. and Wong Staal, F. (1986). Detection of lymphocytes expressing HIV in lymph nodes and peripheral blood from infected individuals by *in situ* hybridisation. *Proc. Natl Acad. Sci. USA* **83**, 772–776.
19. Dalgleish, A.G., Beverley, P.C.L., Clapham, P.C.L., Crawford, D.,

Greaves, M. and Weiss, R.A. (1984). The T4 (CD4) molecule is an essential component of the HIV molecule. *Nature, Lond.* **312**, 763–767.

20. Oldstone, M. (1989). Viruses can cause disease in the absence of morphological evidence of cell injury. *J. Infect. Dis.* **159**, 384–389.

21. Siliciano, R.F., Lawton, T., Knall, C. *et al.* (1988). Analysis of host virus interactions in AIDS with anti-gp120 T cell clones. *Cell* **54**, 561–575.

22. Weinhold, K.Y., Lyerly, H.K., Matthews, T.J. *et al.* (1988). Cellular anti-gp120 cytolyte reactivities in HIV-1 seropositive individuals. *Lancet* **i**, 902–905.

23. Dalgleish, A.G. (1986). The T4 molecule function and structure. *Immunol. Today* **7**, 142–144.

24. Cianacolo, G., Kipuiz, R.J. and Syndermon, R. (1984). Similarity between P15E of murine and feline leukaemia viruses and P12 of HTLV. *Nature, Lond.* **311**, 515–518.

25. Stricker, R., Mcthyly, T., Moody, D.J. *et al.* (1987). An AIDS related cytotoxic auto antibody reacts with a specific antigen on stimulated CD4+ T cells. *Nature, Lond.* **327**, 710–713.

26. Wigzell, H. (1989). Immunopathogenesis of HIV infection. *J. AIDS* **1**, 359–365.

27. Ratner, L., Polmer, S.H., Paul, N. and Ruddle, N. (1987). Cytotoxic factors secreted by cells infected with HIV-1. *AIDS Res. Hum. Retroviruses* **3**, 147–51.

28. Homsy, J., Tateno, M. and Levy, J.A. (1988). Antibody dependent enhancement of HIV-1 infection. *Lancet* **i**, 1285–1286.

29. Lifson, J.D., Fainberg, M.B. and Reyes, G.R. (1986). Induction of CD4 dependent fusion by the HIV envelope protein. *Nature, Lond.* **323**, 725–728.

30. Folks, T.M., Justement, J., Kinter, A., Orenstein, J., Poli, G. and Fauci, A.S. (1988). Characterisation of a premonocyte clone chronically infected with HIV and inducible by PMA. *J. Immunol.* **140**, 1117–1122.

31. Dalgleish, A.G., Chanh, T.C., Kennedy, R.C., Gonda, P., Clapham, P. and Weiss, R.A. (1988). Neutralisation of diverse HIV-1 strains by monoclonal antibodies raised against gp41 peptide. *Virology* **165**, 209–216.

32. Willey, R.L., Ross, E.K., Buckler-White, A.J., Theodore, T.S. and Martin, M.A. (1989). Functional interaction of constant and variable domains of HIV-1 gp120. *J. Virol.* **63**, 3595–3600.

33. Maddon, P.J., Dalgleish, A.G., McDougal, J.S., Clapman, P., Weiss, R.A. and Axel, R. (1986). The T4 gene encodes the AIDS virus receptor and is expressed in the immune system and the brain. *Cell* **47**, 333–348.

34. Hildreth, J.E.K. and Orentas, R.J. (1989). Involvement of LFA-1 in HIV induced synergism formations. *Science* **244**, 1075–1078.

35. Spickett, G. and Dalgleish, A.G. (1988). Cellular immunology of HIV infection. *Clin. Exp. Immunol.* **71**, 1–7.

36. Lasky, L.A., Nakamura, G.M., Smith, D.H. *et al.* (1987). Delineation of a region of HIV-1 gp120 glycoprotein critical for interaction with the CD4 receptor. *Cell* **50**, 975–985.

37. Gelderblom, H.R. and Ozel Pauli, G. (1989). Morphogenesis and morphology of HIV structure–function relations. *Arch. Virol.* **106**, 1–13.

38. Gay, D., Maddon, P., Sekaly, R. *et al.* (1987). Functional interaction between human T cell protein CD4 and HLA-DR antigen. *Nature, Lond.* **328**, 626–628.

39. Diamond, D.C., Sleckman, B.P., Gregory, T., Lasky, L.A., Greenstein, J.L. and Burakoff, S.J. (1988). Inhibition of CD4+ T cell function by the HIV envelope protein gp120. *J. Immunol.* **141**, 3715–3717.

40. Shalaby, M.R., Krowka, J.F., Gregory, T. *et al.* (1987). The effects of HIV recombinant envelope glycoprotein on immune cell functions *in vitro. Cell. Immunol.* **110**, 140–148.

41. Krowka, J., Stites, D., Mills, H. *et al.* (1988). Effects of IL-2 and gp120 of HIV on lymphocyte proliferative responses to CMV. *Clin. Exp. Immunol.* **72**, 179–182.

42. Mittler, R.S. and Hoffmann, M.K. (1989). Synergism between HIV gp120 and gp120 specific antibody in blocking human T cell activation. *Science* **245**, 1380–1382.

43. Manca, F., Habeshaw, J. and Dalgleish, A.G. (1990). The HIV envelope inhibits specific antigen T cell responses by interaction with the memory T cell and not the antigen presenting cell and is prevented by soluble CD4. *Lancet* **i, 335**, 811–815.

44. Mann, D.L., Lusane, F., Popoviz, M. *et al.* (1987). HIV gp120 suppresses PHA-induced lymphocyte blastogenesis. *J. Immunol.* **138**, 2640–2648.

45. Ashwell, J.D. and Schwartz, R.H. (1986). T cell recognition of antigen and Ia molecule as a ternary complex. *Nature, Lond.* **320**, 176–179.

46. Sette, A., Buus, S., Colon, S. *et al.* (1987). Structural characteristics of an antigen required for its interaction with Ia recognition by T cells. *Nature, Lond.* **328**, 395–399.

47. Doyle, C. and Strominger, J.L. (1987). Interaction between CD4 and MHC class II molecules mediates cell adhesion. *Nature, Lond.* **330**, 256–259.

48. Saizawa, K., Rojo, J. and Janeway, C.A. (1987). Evidence for a physical association of CD4 and the CD3 α β T cell receptor. *Nature, Lond.* **328**, 260–263.

49. Linette, G.P., Hatzman, R., Ledbetter, J.A. and June, L.H. (1989). HIV-1 infected T cells show a selective signalling defect after perturbation of CD3 antigen receptor. *Science* **241**, 573–577.

50. Pinching, A., Weiss, R.A. and Miller, D. (1988). AIDS and HIV infection: new perspectives. *Br. Med. Bull.* **44**, 1–19.

51. Shearer, G.M., Bernstein, D.C., Tung, K.S.K. *et al.* (1986). A model for the selective loss of MHC self restricted T cell immune responses during the development of AIDS. *J. Immunol.* **137**, 2514–2521.

52. Shearer, G. (1983). AIDS on consequential of allogeneic 1a antigen recognition. *Immunol. Today* **4**, 181–184.

53. Habeshaw, J. and Dalgleish, A.G. (1989). The relevance of HIV ENV/CD4 interactions to the pathogenesis of acquired immune deficiency syndrome. *J. AIDS* **2**, 457–468.

54. Clouse, K.A., Powell, D., Washington, I., Poli, G. and Strebel, K. (1989). Monokine regulation of HIV-1 expression in a chronically infected human T cell clone. *J. Immunol.* **142**, 431–483.

55. Matsuyama, T., Hamamoto, Y., Kobayashi, S., Kurimoto, M. and Minowada, T. (1988). Enhancement of HIV production by natural lymphotoxin. *Med. Microbiol. Immunol.* **177**, 181–187.

56. Folks, T.M., Jusstement, J., Kiuter, A., Drivarello, C.A. and Fauci, A.S. (1987). Cytokine induced expression of HIV-I LTR by T cell mitogens and the transactivation of HTLV-I. *Science* **238**, 800–802.

57. Vyakaram, A., McKeating, J., Meager, A. and Beverley, P.C.L. (1990). Tumour Necrosis Factor (α,β) induced by HIV-I in peripheral blood mononuclear cells potentiates virus replication. *AIDS* **4**, 21–28.
58. Malkovsky, M., Sondel, P.M., Strober, W. and Dalgleish, A.G. (1988). The Interleukins in acquired disease. *Clin. Exp. Immunol.* **74**, 151–161.
59. Wong, G.H.W., Krowka, J.F., Stites, D.P. and Goeddel, D.V. (1988). *In vitro* anti-HIV activities of TNF and IFN. *J. Immunol.* **140**, 120–124.
60. Folks, T.M., Justement, J., Kinter, A., Dinarello, C.A. and Fauci, A.S. (1987). Cytokine-induced expression of HIV-1 in a chronically infected promonocyte cell line. *Science* **238**, 800–802.
61. Gendelman, H.E., Orenstein, J.M., Martin, M.A. *et al.* (1988). Efficient isolation and propagation of human immunodeficiency virus on recombinant colony stimulating factor I-treated monocytes. *J. Exp. Med.* **167**, 1428–1441.
62. Koyanagi, Y., O'Brien, W.A., Zhao, U.Q., Golde, D.W., Gasson, J.C. and Chen, I.S.Y. (1988). Cytokines alter production of HIV-1 from primary mononuclear phagocytes. *Science* **241**, 1673–1675.
63. Ensoli, B., Nakamura, S., Salahuddin, Z. *et al.* (1989). AIDS Kaposi sarcoma-derived cells express cytokines with autocrine and paracrine growth effects. *Science* **243**, 223–226.
64. Grimaldi, L.M.E., Roos, R.O., Devare, S.G. *et al.* (1988). Restricted heterogeneity of antibody to gp120 and p24 in AIDS. *J. Immunol.* **141**, 114–117.
65. Khalife, J., Guy, B., Lapron, M. *et al.* (1988). Isotypic restriction of the antibody response to HIV. *AIDS Res. Human Retrovirus* **4**, 3–9.
66. Papadopoulos, N.M., Lane, H.C. and Costello, R. (1985). Oligo clonal bands in patients with AIDS. *Clin. Immunol. Immunopathol.* **35**, 43–46.
67. Mills, K., Nixon, D.F. and McMichael, A. (1989). MHC restricted T cell responses to HIV proteins. *AIDS* **3**(S), 101–110.
68. Clapham, P.R., Weber, J.N., Whitby, D. *et al.* (1989). Soluble CD4 blocks the infectivity of diverse strains of HIV and SIV for T cells and monocytes but not for brain and muscle cells. *Nature, Lond.* **337**, 368–370.
69. De Giorgi, L., Povey, S., Habeshaw, J.A. and Matossian-Rogers, A. (1990). Reduction of graft-versus-host disease in neonatal F_1 hybrid mice by preimmunisation of the mother with paternal spleen cells. *Clin. Exp. Immunol.* **79**, 130–134.
70. Dalgleish, A.G., Wilks, D., Walker, L. and Habeshaw, J. (1990). The anti-idiotype approach to designing an AIDS vaccine. In *Vaccines for Sexually Transmitted Diseases*. (Meheus, A. and Spier, R., eds), London, Butterworths. pp. 257–263.

7 | The Biology of the Human T-Lymphotropic Viruses Types 1 and 2 (HTLV-1, HTLV-2)

THOMAS F. SCHULZ

Institute for Cancer Research, Fulham Road, London SW3 6BJ, UK

JONATHAN WEBER

Royal Postgraduate Medical School, Hammersmith Hospital, Ducane Road, London W12 0HS, UK

7.1 INTRODUCTION

While the human immunodeficiency virus (HIV) has attracted the greatest attention since 1982, owing to its rapid pandemic spread and the high mortality of those infected with it, the older, endemic human T-lymphotropic viruses (HTLV) have been relatively neglected. The widespread geographical distribution of HTLV-1, and to a lesser extent HTLV-2, suggests that these agents are of some considerable antiquity as human pathogens. After an enthusiastic period of sero-epidemiology in 1982–1984, many of the details of the distribution and transmission of HTLV around the world still remain obscure or unproven. However, there are enough data on the distribution of these human retroviruses to believe that there are currently more subjects infected by HTLV-1 in the UK than are infected by HIV-1. The HTLV viruses are transmitted both vertically, probably through maternal milk, and horizontally, by blood transfusion and to a lesser degree through sexual intercourse. After long periods of latency, the HTLV viruses are causally associated with a form of acute leukaemia termed the adult T-cell leukaemia (ATL), and with a progressive form of lower limb paralysis known for historical reasons as tropical spastic paraparesis (TSP).

7.2 THE HISTORY OF THE HTLVs

The discovery of human retroviruses belongs firmly to the 1980s, and may come to be seen in the future as one of the most important biological events of the decade. However, the background to the emergence of these much sought after viruses came from more basic cancer research in

AIDS AND THE NEW VIRUSES
ISBN 0–12–200740–9

the 1970s [1, 2]. Through that decade, Gallo and others generated the techniques required for the long-term culture of human lymphocytes, through the discovery of the T cell growth factor (TCGF, now reclassified as interleukin-2, IL-2) [1, 2]. Eventually, one of the many transformed T cell lines derived from human leukaemia and lymphomas generated by Gazdar and given to Gallo's laboratory and others was found in 1980 to contain a novel retrovirus, unrelated to any known animal virus, which was subsequently termed the human T cell leukaemia/lymphoma virus (HTLV) [3]. The patient from which this virus was isolated had been originally diagnosed as having the cutaneous T cell lymphoma, Mycosis fungoides; this was to prove a misdiagnosis. In parallel with Gallo's work, Japanese investigators were studying a newly recognized adult T cell leukaemia (ATL) found in Japan [4]. This leukaemia had been recognized in Japan only 10 years previously, and had been noticed to have a geographical distribution with clustering which suggested a possible infectious aetiology. Cell lines had been derived from peripheral blood lymphocytes from ATL-affected patients by Miyoshi, and were shown by Hinuma to express an antigen (ATL-antigen) which was recognized by antibodies found in all ATL patients' serum [5]. Miyoshi [6] and others showed that there was a novel retrovirus in these cell lines derived from ATL. It was this virus, the ATL-virus reported in 1981, that was responsible for producing the ATL-antigen phenomenon [7]. It was subsequently shown in 1984 to be identical to the human T-leukaemia/ lymphoma virus published by Gallo's group [8]. The final turn of the wheel led to the original patient from which Gallo had isolated HTLV being reclassified as a case of ATL. In 1982, a related virus termed HTLV-2 was isolated from a patient with T cell hairy cell leukaemia [9]; this virus is close to HTLV-1 and serologically cross-reacts in the *gag* and *pol* gene products. One more isolate of HTLV-2 from atypical hairy cell leukaemia has been made [10]. The role of this virus in the causation of a rare T cell variant of hairy cell leukaemia is still uncertain, but it is clear that the very great majority of hairy cell leukaemia cases are of B cell or null cell phenotype, and are not associated with HTLV-2. As the two HTLV-2 isolates come from T cell tumours, these may more closely resemble the HTLV-1 associated malignancies. Owing to difficulty with definitive HTLV-2 diagnosis, it is still unclear whether HTLV-2 is associated causally with any human disease.

An animal virus homologous to HTLV-1 in morphology, antigenicity and genome organization has been isolated from Asian Old World primates (macaques) [11], and subsequently from diverse species of African Old World monkeys and the chimpanzee, but not from any New World species [12, 13]. This has been classified as simian T-lymphotropic virus type 1, STLV-1, and as yet is not associated with clinical disease in infected animals. (The only other animal C-type retrovirus with a genome organization similar to HTLV-1/HTLV-2 is bovine leukaemia virus (see below). This virus is less closely related to HTLV-1 than is STLV-1 [25].)

7.3 VIROLOGICAL ASPECTS

On the basis of electron micrographs HTLV-1 and -2 are classified as C-type retroviruses [2]. In *in vitro* culture they are usually grown in immortalized cell lines, mostly of T cell phenotype, which are obtained by culturing patient cells in the presence of phytohaemagglutinin A (PHA) and IL-2. Most HTLV-1 producing cell lines have been obtained in this way. It is rather difficult to infect established HTLV-1− cell lines with HTLV-1 and -2 *in vitro*. As HTLV-1 and -2 are highly cell-associated viruses which give rise to only very low virus titres in cell culture supernatants [14], this has to be done by extensive co-cultivation using irradiated HTLV producer cell lines. In this way it has been possible to transmit the HTLV-1 to cell lines of non-T lineage and to demonstrate that the virus replicates in a fibrosarcoma (HT 1080) and an osteosarcoma cell line (HOS) [14], as well as in human endothelial cells [15, 16]. Co-cultivation of an HTLV-1 producer cell line with suitable susceptible cell lines produces easily recognizable syncytia [17, 18]. This observation has been exploited to demonstrate that HTLV-1 envelope proteins must bind to membrane molecules present in a wide variety of cells, both of human and non-human origin [17]. To circumvent the experimental difficulties posed by the cell-associated nature of HTLV, HTLV/VSV pseudotype viruses were produced [19]. These "pseudotypes" consist of the core of vesicular stomatitis virus (VSV) and the envelope of HTLV-1 or -2, and therefore have the host range of the latter, are lytic in tissue culture and produce an easily recognizable cytopathic effect because of their VSV core, and can be obtained as cell-free virus in reasonable titres [19, 20, 21]. Using this approach, it has been shown that the cellular receptor for HTLV-1 is also the receptor for HTLV-2, and that it is expressed on a wide variety of human cells as well as on cells from some non-human species (simian, canine, feline, mink, rabbit, hamster and rat cells) [19, 20, 22]. Therefore, the apparent T cell tropism of HTLV-1 and -2 observed *in vivo* does not seem to be determined at the receptor level. Whether HTLV-1 can also replicate *in vivo* in cells of non-T cell lineage, as observed *in vitro* [14–16], is not quite clear at present. Studies in transgenic mice to be discussed below indicate that control regions of the virus genome (the LTRs) are active in cells of mesenchymal origin and in the thymus, and that this may contribute to the tropism of HTLV-1. By testing the infectivity of HTLV-1/VSV pseudotype viruses for somatic cell hybrids between mouse and human cells the gene coding for the receptor of HTLV could be mapped to chromosome 17 [22].

The envelope proteins of HTLV-1 and -2 are also the target of neutralizing antibodies [17, 19, 21]. Neutralizing antibodies inhibit syncytia formation as well as the infectivity of HTLV/VSV pseudotypes [17, 19, 21]. These assays can therefore be used to measure the level of neutralizing antibodies in patient sera [17, 19, 20]. From these studies it emerged that Japanese as well as American HTLV-1 isolates are neutralized to the same extent by sera of Japanese, American and British patients. This indicates that neutralizing epitopes of HTLV-1 represent a single serotype world-wide [21]. In contrast, these neutralization assays can be used to differentiate between antibodies to HTLV-1 and HTLV-2 and thus to discriminate serologically between these two viruses [19, 20].

7.4   MOLECULAR BIOLOGY

7.4.1   Genome organization

The genomic organization of HTLV-1 [23, 24] has the characteristic features of a typical retroviral genome, i.e. the three open reading frames representing the *gag*, *pol* and *env* genes coding for the nucleocapsid proteins, the three retroviral enzymes reverse transcriptase, proteinase and integrase, and the two membrane proteins, respectively. As in any typical replication-competent retrovirus, the genome is flanked by two long terminal repeats (LTRs) which contain promoter and enhancer functions essential for the transcription of viral genes (see Section 7.4.2). Another feature of a retroviral genome, the packaging site, i.e. the short stretch of genomic sequence that is essential for the binding of genomic RNA to capsid proteins as a prerequisite for the packaging of viral RNA, has not been mapped in HTLV-1.

In addition to these features, which are typical for most retroviruses, HTLV-1 has additional genes coding for two regulatory proteins named *rex* and *tax*, as well as a third protein, p21, of as yet unknown function (see below). These genes are localized downstream of the envelope gene (Fig. 7.1). Among animal retroviruses similar genes are only found in the close relatives of HTLV-1, bovine leukaemia virus (BLV) [25] and simian T-lymphotropic virus 1 (STLV-1) [26] but not in other C-type retroviruses. Genes with very similar functions are also found in some members of the lentivirus family such as HIV and SIV [27, 28].

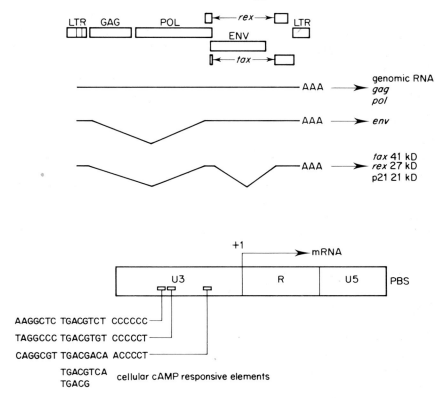

Fig. 7.1 Schematic representation of the HTLV-1 genome, its transcription pattern and the structure of the HTLV-1 LTR. The top third of the figure depicts the genome organization and the position of different genes discussed in the text. The middle third of the figure represents the splicing pattern of the most important mRNAs transcribed from this genome, and on the right of the arrows are listed the viral proteins translated from the respective messenger RNAs. The bottom of the figure indicates the position of th U3, R and U5 regions of the HTLV-1 LTR, the beginning of the transcription which defines the 5′ end of R, and the three octanucleotide sequences in the U3 region and their homology to other cellular cAMP responsive elements (see text). PBS: primer binding site.

7.4.2 Long terminal repeats

As in every retrovirus, the two identical long terminal repeats, abbreviated LTRs, which flank the virus genome on either side, contain the promoter and enhancer sequences necessary for viral transcription as well as elements necessary for the proper processing of viral transcripts, e.g. the polyadenylation site, and for integration into cellular DNA. By convention they are subdivided into U5, R, and U3 regions (Fig. 7.1). The U3 region contains the enhancer and promoter elements of a retrovirus. Three imperfect 21 base-pair repeats localized in U3 have been shown to be required for the promoter function of the U3 region of HTLV-1 [29, 30]. These repeats contain a core pentanucleotide TGACG, which is also found in some cellular genes and is thought to represent a cAMP responsive element [31]. They are essential for the effect of the HTLV-1 transactivator, *tax*, on the HTLV-1 LTR (see below). Cellular DNA binding factors interacting with these repeats have been characterized [32]. In addition, raised intracellular cAMP levels enhance transcription from the viral LTR [32]. These findings indicate that certain cellular DNA binding factors involved in controlling transcription from normal cellular genes also act on and control transcription from the viral LTR and that, more specifically, HTLV-1 may exploit control mechanisms involved in the cAMP regulatory pathway.

From earlier work on murine retroviruses, it is known that the U3 region may also — at least to a certain extent — determine the cell tropism of a retrovirus. In spite of the wide distribution of its receptor (see above), HTLV-1 seems to replicate only in a limited number of cell types. After introduction into the germline of transgenic mice the HTLV-1 LTR seemed to be active in thymus, muscle, and possibly other mesenchymal tissues [33–35]. Because of this tissue-specific expression the HTLV-1 LTR may, like the LTR of murine retroviruses, be at least partially responsible for the observed tropism of HTLV-1 and -2.

The second compartment within the LTR, termed R, is defined as a sequence which is found at both ends of the genomic RNA of a retrovirus. Figure 7.1 illustrates how transcription of a DNA provirus, which is flanked by complete LTRs on both ends, results in a genomic transcript starting with the R sequence at the 5′ end and terminating in a poly A tail at the 3′ end. The beginning of R is therefore defined by the 5′ end of both genomic and subgenomic mRNAs. This R sequence is much longer in HTLV-1 (229 bp) than in most other retroviruses (usually 20–80 bp, 97 bp in HIV-1, 173 bp in HIV-2) [23, 27, 36]. In addition, it lacks a polyadenylation signal (AATAAA) that is normally found 10–30 bp upstream of the end of R (the 3′ end of the R sequence at the right-hand side of the genome corresponds to the end of the genomic RNA before addition of the poly A tail — see Fig. 7.1). Such a polyadenylation signal is, however, found within the U3 region and is thus located 276 bp upstream of the site where the poly A tail has to be added during processing of a genomic transcript. This has led to the suggestion that parts of U3 and the complete R present in the genomic RNA may form a hairpin loop, which would bring the polyadenylation site in U3 and the site of poly A addition closer together [23]. As such a loop could not be formed on the 5′ end of the genomic RNA (because of the lack of U3), this could be one possible way to explain why genomic transcripts are only processed at the 3′ end of the genome.

The R region also contains the splice donor, which is involved in generating the two subgenomic messenger RNAs giving rise to the envelope and control proteins (see below and Fig. 7.1) [37]. The donor for these splicing events is located at bp 471 and contained in the sequence AGGUAAG. This sequence is identical in HTLV-2 and BLV and highly conserved in STLV (GGGUAAG) [37].

7.4.3 Gag–pol

The first major open reading frame of the HTLV-1 genome codes for a *gag* precursor of 429aa that is cleaved into the three typical *gag* proteins of a retrovirus. These have molecular weights of 19 kD, 24 kD and 15 kD [38–40]. The carboxyterminal p15 represents the nucleic acid-binding protein. A duplicated sequence in p15 is highly homologous to a similar region in bovine leukaemia virus and therefore thought to be of functional importance [25].

The second major open reading frame within the *gag–pol* complex codes for the proteinase of HTLV-1. This reading frame partially overlaps with that of *gag* [24]. HTLV-1 proteinase is generated from the full length genomic mRNA by frameshift suppression of the *gag* terminator codon. This frameshift occurs in a stretch of six A residues located close to the end of the *gag* gene and results in a *gag–proteinase* fusion protein of approximately 76 kD which is then cleaved into the *gag* components p19, p24, p15 and the free proteinase [41].

The reverse transcriptase of HTLV-1 is encoded by a different open reading frame that codes for a 99 kD protein [23]. A protein of this size is present in HTLV-1 expressing cell lines [42]. The reverse transcriptase of HTLV-I prefers Mg^{2+} as a divalent cation [42].

7.4.4 Env

The envelope reading frame has the capacity to code for a protein of 481 amino acids [23, 24]. After glycosylation, the envelope precursor has a molecular weight of 62 kD and is processed by proteolytic cleavage to yield an outer envelope protein of 46 kD and a transmembrane protein of 21 kD [38, 43]. The envelope precursor is translated from a 4.2 kb mRNA in which the *gag* region and most of the *pol* region have been spliced out (see Fig. 7.1). The donor for this splicing event is at bp 471 in the R region of the 5′ LTR, as outlined above. The corresponding splice acceptor is localized in the *pol* gene at position 4993, 187 bp upstream of the *env* initiator codon. The sequence immediately preceding the splice acceptor, UAUUUCAAG, is closely related to a similar sequence in BLV (UCAUUUCAG) and identical to one in STLV. The equivalent region in HTLV-2 is more distantly related (UCCCUCCAG) [37]. The initiator codon of the *env* gene is located 5 bp upstream of the termination codon of the *pol* gene [23, 24].

(a) *Function of envelope proteins*

The envelope proteins of HTLV-1 mediate the binding of the virus to its receptor on the cell surface. This follows from the observation that pseudotype viruses carrying an HTLV-1 envelope can bind to cells as outlined earlier in Section 7.3. By analogy with other retroviruses, in particular HIV, one would expect the outer envelope protein of HTLV-1, gp46, to be responsible for the attachment of the virus to cells.

The envelope proteins of HTLV are also the target of neutralizing antibodies [17, 19, 21]. Cynomologous monkeys and rabbits immunized with recombinant envelope proteins produce neutralizing antibodies and are protected from challenge with HTLV-1 [44, 45]. Although there is some serological cross-reactivity between the envelopes of HTLV-1 and -2, neutralizing antibodies seem to be specific for either of the two viruses [19, 20], as mentioned earlier. Some of the epitopes eliciting anti-envelope antibodies in humans have been localized and are found both on gp46 and gp21. Three synthetic peptides corresponding to amino acids 190–209, 296–312 and 374–392 reacted with many, but not all, human HTLV-1 sera tested [46]. The localization of those epitopes that form the target of neutralizing antibodies has not yet been determined. In the case of BLV, a relative of HTLV-1, neutralizing antibodies have been found to be directed at non-linear, conformational epitopes [47]. It is therefore possible that conformational epitopes are also important for the neutralizing antibody response to HTLV-1. In addition, one linear neutralizing epitope of BLV [48] shows homology with one of the reported antigenic epitopes of HTLV-1 [46]. Whether this HTLV-1 epitope is also the target for neutralizing antibodies in humans is at present under investigation.

The transmembrane protein, gp21, contains a sequence near its amino terminus which has been implicated in immunosuppression. The transmembrane proteins of several retroviruses (FeLV, RLV) have been shown to inhibit lymphocyte proliferation and macrophage function *in vitro* [49]. A synthetic peptide derived from a region homologous (but not identical) between the p15E of MoLV, FeLV and the gp21 of HTLV-1 inhibited lymphocyte proliferation *in vitro* [50]. The importance of these findings for immunodeficiency states sometimes associated with HTLV-1 infections is not clear at present.

7.4.5 pX

The fifth genomic region, often referred to as pX, is localized between the 3' end of the *env* gene and the 3' LTR. A similar region has been identified in HTLV-2, BLV, and STLV. It contains at least four short open reading frames termed pX-I, pX-II, pX-III and pX-IV [23]. A possible fifth reading frame has recently been noted in this region [24]. This region codes for three proteins of HTLV-1, termed *tax*, *rex* and p21. The functions of *tax* and *rex* have been elucidated and these proteins have been shown to represent important control proteins essential for the life-cycle of the virus. The function of p21 is unknown at present. All three proteins are translated from a doubly spliced 2.1 kb mRNA as shown in Fig. 7.1 [37, 51–56].

The first splicing event is similar to the one used to generate the 4.2 kb *env* mRNA, whereas the second splicing event joins the *env* initiator codon ATG and the following residue with a splice acceptor within the pX region. The splice donor for the second splicing event is contained in the sequence G<u>G</u>GUAAG (splice donor underlined). As for the first splicing event, the sequences surrounding the splice donors and acceptors are conserved in the HTLV/STLV/BLV family and this particular sequence is identical in BLV and STLV whereas in HTLV-2 it is changed in one position (G<u>G</u>GUAAU). The splice acceptor for this second splice event is localized at nucleotide 7301 at the end of the sequence UAUUAUCAG. Again, this sequence is completely conserved in STLV and somewhat more divergent in HTLV-2 and BLV [37].

For *tax*, translation of this doubly spliced messenger RNA starts at the initiator codon of the *env*; then, because of the second splicing event, it proceeds in the pX-IV reading frame of the pX region (see Fig. 7.1). This generates a protein of 40 kD. For *rex*, translation starts 56 nucleotides upstream of the *env* initiator codon in the *pol* gene and proceeds in a different reading frame from *tax*. The *rex* reading frame corresponds to the pX-III reading frame but extends the latter at the 5' end by 78 amino acids. This yields a protein of 27 kD which has no amino acid homology with *tax*. The third protein translated from this polycystronic messenger RNA, p21, is produced from the same reading frame as *rex* with translation starting 78 amino acids downstream and is thus a shortened form of *rex* which corresponds exactly to the pX-III reading frame [52].

(a) *Function of* tax

The *tax* protein activates transcription from the HTLV-1 LTR and is therefore an important regulator of viral replication [54–60]. In addition, *tax* has been shown to enhance the transcription of some cellular genes such as those for interleukin 2 (IL-2), the IL-2 receptor (IL-2R), IL-3, IL-4, granulocyte–macrophage colony-stimulating factor, and c-fos [61–69]. The *tax* protein has been shown to be localized in the nucleus of the cell, which is consistent with its function [70].

Tax acts on the U3 region of the LTR in an indirect manner. The U3 region contains three copies of an imperfectly conserved 21 base-pair sequence. Two or more copies of this 21 bp motif, regardless of orientation, can serve as a sufficient target for transactivation of the LTR by *tax* [29, 30, 71, 72]. However, some cellular genes that can also be activated by *tax* lack this sequence motif, indicating that the latter is not an absolute requirement for *tax*-mediated transactivation. In fact, evidence available at present would suggest that *tax* does not interact directly with target sequences in the LTR, but that it induces the expression of cellular factors which may then in turn activate the LTR or cellular genes.

Specifically, several nuclear proteins have been identified which seem to be induced by *tax* and which bind to the 21 bp repeats in the LTR [32]. In addition, other *tax*-inducible factors have been found which bind to the $\varkappa$-B sequence motif in the IL-2 receptor α-chain enhancers, thus increasing the expression of this molecule in T cells. The same factor is normally expressed upon stimulation of T cells by mitogen and it therefore seems that *tax* can exploit and interact with cellular pathways of activation [73, 74]. Apart from the IL-2 receptor α-chain, HTLV-1-expressing human T cells also express platelet derived growth factor (PDGF) and CR2, the receptor for the C3d fragment of human complement component C3 and Epstein–Barr virus [75–77]. Although it has not formally been established in the case of PDGF and CR2 that this is due to the action of *tax*, this is likely. *Tax* would therefore resemble other transactivating viral proteins like the adenovirus E1a, the SV40 large T antigen and herpes virus immediate-early proteins, all of which transactivate many different cellular genes (for review, see [78]). Whether *tax*, like adenovirus E1a, also physically interacts with cellular factors presumed to be important in regulating cell growth (for a review, see [79]), is unknown at present.

Introduced into transgenic mice under the control of the HTLV-1 LTR, *tax* is expressed in muscle and thymus [33, 34], leading to the appearance of mesenchymal tumours and thymic atrophy. Some of these tumours resemble human neurofibromas [35] and arise from peripheral nerve sheaths. These findings show that *tax* has transforming properties *in vivo*. Whether these observations can shed light on the pathogenesis of human neurofibromas (van Recklinghausen's disease) is uncertain.

It is of interest to highlight that a similar transactivating protein found in HIV, *tat*, differs in its mode of action. A region downstream of the cap site in R, *tar*, is important for the action of HIV-*tat* which exerts its transcription-enhancing effect by binding to the nascent RNA [80, 81]. So far, no clear-cut evidence for an effect of HIV-*tat* on cellular genes has been reported.

(b) *Function of* rex

Analysis of the function of *rex* has revealed a novel mechanism of controlling gene expression. *Rex*, a phosphoprotein also localized in the nucleus [52], acts on the viral RNA transcripts within a region in the 3′ LTR (within base pairs 302 and 560) [82]. This prevents the primary transcript from being spliced into its subgenomic mRNAs yielding the envelope, *tax*, *rex* and 21 kd protein [83]. This mode of action is similar to that of the analogous HIV protein, *rev*, except that the *rev*-responsive region is localized within the sequence coding for the transmembrane protein, gp41. *Rex* can substitute for HIV-1 *rev in vitro* [84], although there is no significant sequence homology between *rex* and *rev*. As *rev* has been shown to inhibit splicing by activating the nuclear export of unspliced viral messenger RNAs [85], it is possible that *rex* acts in a similar manner.

The level of *rex* protein therefore determines the degree to which full-length genomic RNA or spliced RNA yielding the control proteins are made, and *rex* can therefore be regarded as a "molecular switch". In the presence of sufficient levels of *rex* the balance would be tilted towards generating full-length genomic RNA and the structural proteins, thus facilitating the production of new virus, whereas in the absence of *rex* a shift in favour of producing the control genes *tax* and *rex* would occur. Increased levels of *tax* would then, in turn, enhance transcription from the LTR (as well as acting on cellular genes). This would at first lead to increasing levels of *tax* and *rex* until sufficient *rex* levels would have accumulated to tilt the balance in favour of production of structural proteins and also to inhibit a further accumulation of *tax*, thus controlling the effect of *tax* on viral transcription.

So far there is no evidence to indicate that *rex* may act on cellular RNAs in a similar manner.

7.5   MOLECULAR PATHOGENESIS OF HTLV-1 INFECTIONS

As will be discussed in detail below, there are two main diseases that have been associated with HTLV-1 — adult T cell leukaemia (ATL) and tropical spastic paraparesis (TSP). HTLV-2 has been isolated occasionally from patients with hairy cell leukaemia of T cell lineage, but its causal association with this disease remains uncertain. The following paragraph summarizes what is known at present about the pathogenic mechanisms involved in HTLV-1-induced disease.

7.5.1   Adult T cell leukaemia/lymphoma (ATL)

From a number of *in vitro* studies it is clear that HTLV-1 can immortalize human T cells into permanently growing *in vitro* cell lines [6, 86, 87]. The binding of HTLV-1 to its receptor on human peripheral blood T cells induces a short-lived proliferation in a subpopulation of T cells [88]. This phenomenon can be obtained with inactivated virus and has nothing to do with the eventual immortalization that some of these cells undergo at a later stage. Inducing an invaded cell to proliferate may be of advantage to an invading retrovirus, as some of the steps in the retroviral life-cycle, e.g. integration into the host cell genome, probably only occur in a dividing cell. Interestingly, there is an analogy to another transforming virus, Epstein Barr virus (EBV). The EBV receptor on B cells, CR2 (CD21), when cross-linked by antibodies or by its natural ligand, the complement fragment C3d, can induce a B cell proliferation by allowing pre-activated B cells to proceed through the S-phase of their cycle [89–91]. Too little is known at present about the identity of the HTLV-1 receptor to know how closely related the initial processes induced by these two transforming viruses are.

After entering the cell, HTLV-1 follows the normal steps of a retroviral life-cycle: uncoating, reverse transcription of the genomic RNA and integration into the host genome. In the case of HTLV-1 the integration is random, i.e. there is no predilection for certain sites in the genome [92]. The analysis of integrated HTLV-1 genomes in leukaemic cells indicates that many of the integrated genomes are defective [24, 93]. In most cases, however, the pX region, coding for *tax* and *rex*, is retained along with the 5′ LTR [24]. Whether these deletions eliminating large parts of the viral genome occur when HTLV-1 is integrated in the cell genome for the first time, or whether they occur and/or are selected for at a later stage of the transformation process is unknown.

Although immortalized T cell lines and ATL cells have some common features, in particular the high level of IL-2 receptor α-chain molecules [94], they also differ in several important respects. In *in vitro* immortalized T cells the viral genome is transcribed and virus-encoded proteins, among them the structural *gag* and *envelope* proteins as well as *tax*, are expressed. Apart from the IL-2 receptor, these cells may also express other cellular genes, e.g. secrete IL-2 or platelet-derived growth factor (PDGF), or express CR2 as indicated above. In contrast, ATL cells, when examined either in biopsy specimens or before *in vitro* culture, usually do not transcribe the HTLV-1 genome, and therefore do not express viral proteins, in particular no transforming *tax* [95]. To explain this apparent discrepancy it is therefore assumed, as with other malignancies, that the generation of malignant ATL cells occurs in several steps. In an initial step (or series of steps) infection of T cells with HTLV-1 would result in a population of oligoclonal T cells that are to some extent no longer subject to normal growth control, but are not yet malignant. These cells would express *tax* as well as other viral proteins and the effect of *tax* on other cellular genes (expression of IL-2R, IL-2 and possibly other growth factors) would result in the proliferation of infected T cells by an autocrine mechanism. The phenotype of these cells would thus be comparable to *in vitro* immortalized T cells. Cells expressing IL-2 receptors as well as viral antigens have been detected in the peripheral blood of seropositive, healthy individuals [96, 146].

However, in order to generate malignant ATL cells, an additional step would seem to be necessary. This step may involve one or more chromosomal abnormalities that are the hallmark of ATL cells, but are not found in *in vitro* immortalized T cells. This chromosomal abnormality is considered to represent the actual transforming event.

There does not seem to be a uniform pattern of chromosomal aberrations in ATL but abnormalities involving chromosome 14q11, carrying the T cell receptor α-chain, as well as chromosomes 3 and 6, seem to be common [97, 98]. The gene locus for a T cell receptor is likely to be an "active" locus in a T cell because of gene rearrangements occurring during normal T cell maturation. It is therefore conceivable that such a gene might be especially prone to "accidents" and that immortalization of a T cell by HTLV-1 might greatly enhance the chance of such an accident occurring. It is less clear why the other gene loci (chromosomes 3 and 6) should be involved with a certain frequency. This scenario bears some resemblance to the pathogenesis of Epstein–Barr virus-associated Burkitt's lymphoma, where chromosomal aberrations involving immunoglobulin loci on chromosomes 2, 14 and 22 have been shown to involve translocation of the *c-myc* oncogene on chromosome 8 under the control of immunoglobulin gene enhancers — for a review see [99]. However, in the case of HTLV-1 it is not clear why the observed chromosomal aberrations should lead to cell transformation. Since the pattern of chromosomal abnormalities in ATL is not as homogenous as in Burkitt's lymphoma, there may be more than one "genetic accident" that can contribute to the emergence of ATL.

In these cells *tax* would no longer be needed and would therefore be switched off, which would explain the experimental findings in ATL cells. If this model is correct, then HTLV-1-induced ATL would be another example of a virus-induced neoplasm where the virus only prepares the stage for the actually transforming event.

7.5.2 Tropical spastic paraparesis (TSP)

In contrast to ATL, where we have an idea about at least some stages in the development of ATL, our knowledge about the pathogenic role of HTLV-1 in TSP is still very limited, although the serological evidence for an involvement of HTLV-1 in this disorder is very good (see below). Peripheral blood lymphocytes of patients with TSP harbour the virus as assessed by the ability to amplify HTLV-1-like sequences by PCR and also to obtain virus-producing cell lines in tissue culture [100–102]. The virus isolates recovered from TSP patients seem to be rather similar to those obtained from ATL cells. Whether minor differences between these isolates can explain the different disease associations is unclear at present. HTLV-1 sequences have also been recovered from the cerebrospinal fluid. However, it is unknown at present what causes the dymyelination observed in TSP lesions. By analogy with morphologically related lesions encountered in animal models of demyelinating diseases, and especially because of the cellular infiltrate observed in these lesions, it is speculated that an autoimmune T cell response may play a role. What the role of HTLV-1 should be in this is a mystery, although it has been proposed that HTLV-1 may expand clones of autoimmune T cells with, for example, an antimyelin specificity.

7.6 SEROLOGY AND SEROEPIDEMIOLOGY

7.6.1 Antigens of HTLV

Replication of HTLV-1 *in vivo* leads to the production of virally encoded structural and regulatory proteins and their precursors, many of which are antigenic [38, 103]. The structural genes *gag*, *pol* and *env* encode three precursor proteins, which are the major antigens used to define antibodies to HTLV-1, and hence infection [104]. The structural proteins of HTLV-1, all of which are antigenic and recognized by human antibodies, have been discussed above. The regulatory gene products *tax* and *rex* appear to be antigenic [38, 105], but they are not currently used for routine diagnostic purposes. One recent report describes antibodies to *tax* in seronegative individuals from a group at risk for HTLV-1 infection. These *tax* antibody-positive individuals were also positive for HTLV-1 by PCR (see below) [106].

Table 7.1 HTLV assays.

High sensitivity, low specificity screening assays
Whole virus ELISA
Particle agglutination
Immunofluorescence on HTLV-1 transformed line

Higher specificity, lower sensitivity assays
Competitive ELISA or RIA
Neutralizing antibody
Immunoblot
RIPA

Definitive assays for virus
Culture
PCR

Infection by HTLV leads to an antibody response against structural proteins that is of high titre and persists life-long; this is the basis of the identification of infection in the individual subject, and in populations [104]. As with HIV, the options for diagnosis begin with simple, sensitive and inexpensive serological screening assays such as the ELISA or particle agglutination assay. Progression to assays of greater specificity such as the immunoblot, radioimmuno-precipitation (RIPA) or neutralization assay may be required, and finally molecular assays are being developed, which now mean the amplification of the HTLV genome by the polymerase chain reaction (PCR) (see below), or most laboriously of all, growth of HTLV by cell culture techniques.

(a) *HTLV assays (Table 7.1)*

The commercial screening assays currently in use have antigen derived from cell lysates of HTLV-1-transformed cell lines on the solid phase for the test antibody binding. The assays systems are mostly direct enzyme-linked immunoassays, with the crude virus extract adsorbed onto the solid phase, usually a multititre plate. Binding of test sera are recognized by standard amplification techniques, such as peroxidase or biotin/avidin. Alternatively, there is a commercial gel particle agglutination assay (GPA); this uses the same HTLV-1-transformed cell line adsorbed onto the particles. This assay is the most sensitive, and is widely used for serology.

However, HTLV is a highly cell-associated virus in culture, with little free virus generated into the culture supernatant. This means that the viral antigens are inevitably heavily contaminated with normal lymphocyte antigens. This factor is probably the major cause of non-specific false positivity, where antibodies to lymphocyte antigen are present in the test serum. In some populations, the false positive rate by the GPA assay technique may be as high as 10% [107], and as high as 5% by direct ELISA. As the false positivity is highest in multiparous females, these assays must be interpreted with caution in ante-natal populations, and as discussed further below, the use of ante-natal clinic attenders for seroepidemiology may be misleading. The lymphocyte-based false reactivity in these assays could be most readily overcome by using recombinant antigen on the solid phase. There is considerable activity in this field, with recombinant proteins derived from *Escherichia coli*, baculovirus and chinese hamster ovary (CHO) cells in preparation. However, although these recombinant proteins may yield excellent antigens in the future, they are not currently available, and thus serology must be interpreted in the light of the currently available technology.

In order to increase the specificity of the ELISA assays, two modified assays have been developed. One uses an IgG capture technique that is "cleaner" in abolishing non-specific binding to the solid phase [108]. The other uses a competitive assay, where the test serum has to compete with the standard human antibody to HTLV-1 onto the antigen on the solid phase [109]. Antilymphocytic antibodies tend to have lower avidity for the antigen than anti-HTLV, and so this technique reduces the most common cause of false positivity. However, this assay has a slightly lower sensitivity, and so will probably become a confirmation assay; in addition, this assay format will not pick up antibodies to HTLV-like viruses. The competing antibody should be a human antiserum to HTLV-1, as use of an animal polyclonal antibody to HTLV-1 may give lower specificity [107].

The major dilemma with HTLV serology is the lack of a gold standard for serological reactivity. The immunoblot is most commonly used for definitive HTLV serology, again with cell-derived lysed whole virus preparations blotted onto the nitrocellulose. Human antisera to HTLV-1 from clinical cases generally react with *gag*, *pol* and *env* proteins. Therefore bands are visible strongly at 24 kD, 19 kD and (less commonly) 15 kD; in addition, gp46 and gp21 are seen [107], and there may be precursor *gag*, *env* and *pol* gene products visualized. Figure 7.2 shows the immunoblot reactivity of three subjects infected by HTLV-1 by diverse assays: lane 14 presented with TSP, and has high titre antibody to all viral antigens, including the *env* gene products gp46 and gp21. The case in lane 15 presented with ATL, has definite reactivity against *gag* and *pol* proteins and precursors, but has only faint reactivity against the gp46; this sera neutralized HTLV-1 to a titre of 1:1000, and was positive in the competitive ELISA assay. The case in lane 16 is the wife of lane 15, also neutralized HTLV-1 at 1:1000, and reacted in competitive ELISA; however, this subject has only weak reactivity with *gag* proteins. It is possible that duration of infection leads to broader antigenic re-activity on immunoblot, but this has not been convincingly demonstrated. This discrepancy of reactivity on immunoblot leads to considerable practical problems. Sera which react with only one or two *gag* bands on immunoblot are found increasingly, and in some populations this *gag* reactivity may be the most common serological finding. These sera may be further resolved by radioimmuno-precipitation (RIPA), which enhances the reactivity against the *env* proteins. However, RIPA is a laborious assay, not suited to widespread application. At the moment, these indeterminate reactivities are a considerable problem, particularly for blood transfusion directors, but equally for the subject involved. The solution to these may lie in the application of more diverse assays. Bioassays, such as virus neutralization, may be performed to study further the specificity of the anti-*env* response [19, 20]. Neutralization assays use the high levels (> 1:1000) of virus-neutralizing antibodies generated in HTLV infection; the assays are either infection inhibition assays, using syncytial formation as an end-point, or use a pseudotyped HTLV virus with a lytic virus (such as VSV) as an indirect plaque assay [19, 20]. These assays are highly specific for anti-*env* antibodies to HTLV-1 and HTLV-2, and may help to discriminate true positives from indeterminate *gag*-only reactive sera. However, these bioassays are currently only a research tool.

More recently, the polymerase chain reaction technique has begun to be used for the diagnosis of infections with HTLV-1 and HTLV-2 [101, 102, 106, 110, 111]. In addition to demonstrating the presence of virus-

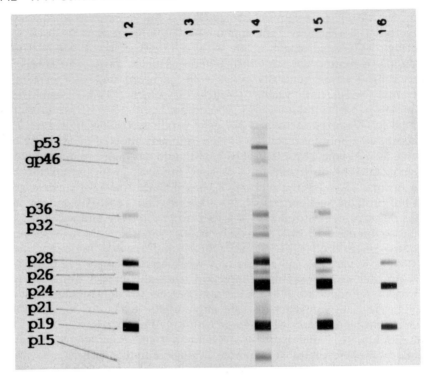

Fig. 7.2   Western blot strips of HTLV-1 stained with representative patient samples showing the position of some typical HTLV-1 bands. Lane 12, positive control; lane 13, negative control; lane 14, patient with tropical spastic paraparesis (TSP); lane 15, patient with adult T cell leukaemia (ATL); lane 16, healthy carrier (wife of 15).

specific nucleic acid sequences in patient samples, this technique allows the subsequent characterization of the amplified DNA by either restriction mapping [110] or sequence analysis [101, 102]. In this way it has been possible to show that patients with TSP harbour HTLV-1 viruses that differ only minimally from isolates obtained from patients with ATL [101, 102]. In the same way it has been possible to amplify and sequence the complete envelope of HTLV-1 from Brazilian ATL cases and to compare the sequence with that of Japanese and Caribbean isolates (M.L. Calabrò, T.F. Schulz and D. Catovsky, unpublished results). Using oligonucleotide primers derived from the *tax* gene, which are capable of amplifying both HTLV-1 and HTLV-2, and subsequent restriction enzyme digestion to differentiate between these two viruses, it was found that the majority of seropositive drug abusers in New Orleans were in fact harbouring HTLV-2 [110]. PCR has also been used to demonstrate HTLV-1 sequences in a lymphoma initially diagnosed as Hodgkin's disease from a seronegative patient [111] and in patients who were seronegative in standard serological assays but had antibodies to the *tax* protein [106]. These examples show that this technique clearly has great potential for the diagnosis of HTLV-related infections, but it is important to stress that at this point in time its reliability has not been sufficiently validated for it to be used as a routine diagnostic test. Questions related to false positive results observed with this extremely sensitive technique have to be addressed systematically and at the moment PCR should still be regarded as a research tool. However, in the future genome detection is likely to be more commonly used; the culture techniques for HTLV are time-consuming, and direct amplification by PCR is most attractive.

(b) *Distinction of HTLV-1 from HTLV-2*

The distinction between HTLV-1 and HTLV-2 infection is currently difficult, as in serological terms they are cross-reactive in whole-virus ELISA and GPA assays. The competitive assay will discriminate HTLV-1 and HTLV-2 in quantitative rather than qualitative terms, and competitive assays for both viruses have been used by Tedder *et al.* [109]. The major limit to a serological distinction has been the lack of a high titre virus-producing HTLV-2 cell line. Sequence homology and antigenic conservation is highest for the *gag* and *pol* genes, similar to HIV-1 and HIV-2 serology. However, there are differnces in the *env* gene, and the viruses appear to have distinct neutralizing epitopes, without cross-neutralization in either direction [19, 20]. Therefore neutralizing antibody assays will distinguish HTLV-1 from HTLV-2, but these assays are highly specialized [19, 20]. As mentioned above, a rapid distinction between HTLV-1 and -2 is possible by PCR [110].

7.6.2 Epidemiology

Given the caveats above as to the problems with serology, and the lack of attention to HTLV owing to the AIDS epidemic, the distribution and transmission are not as reliably known as would be wished. Table 7.2 attempts to list those areas where HTLV-1 is known to exist, associated with adult T-cell leukaemia/lymphoma (ATL) or tropical spastic paraparesis (TSP); areas where seropositivity is reported, but no disease is apparent; and areas where serology results lack confirmation, and no HTLV-associated disease has been reported.

Table 7.2   Distribution of HTLV-1.

Category 1: Definite virus and disease
Japan
Caribbean Islands/Caribbean immigrants to UK and elsewhere
South-eastern USA
West/Central Africa

Category 2: Definite virus, probable disease
East, Central Africa
Eastern Siberia
Colombia/Chile

Category 3: Possible virus, no disease reported
Papua New Guinea/south-west Pacific islands
Other African countries
Australian aboriginals
Eskimo/Inuit/Aleuts
Norway

Category 4: Sporadic/epidemic disease
IV drug users
Homosexual men
Heterosexual partners and children of index cases
Blood transfusion-associated cases
Sporadic case reports in Europe, no risk factors

The distribution of HTLV-1 through south-western Japan and the northern island, Hokkaido [7], and through the Caribbean, is now beyond reasonable doubt [112]. Prevalence ranges from 6–12% in these locations, and the seroprevalence increases with increasing age, suggesting either that transmission is now less common than previously in these areas, or that there is delayed seroconversion to HTLV-1 over time [113], or that horizontal transmission spreads HTLV-1 within cohorts. Despite a report from the Caribbean that Barbados has had a stable epidemiological pattern of HTLV-1 infection over an 18-year period [114], data from Japan suggest that a cohort effect is the likeliest cause of the apparent increase in seroprevalence with age. Ueda shows that cohorts of women born from 1930–1960 have decreasing prevalence of HTLV serology, but that seroprevalence is stable within age cohorts. This suggests that horizontal transmission between subjects was rare, as was delayed seroconversion, and that HTLV-1 is now less common in endemic areas [115]. Other studies from Japan have failed to provide evidence for delayed seroconversion to HTLV-1, during an 18-year follow-up of children born to infected mothers [116].

In the USA, HTLV-1 infection is found in the south-eastern states, in the black population who, one assumes, share the same risk as the Caribbean population. This most likely reflects ancient infection from their origin in West Africa [1]. Testing of blood donors in the USA shows rates of between 0 and 0.1%, depending on geographical location [117]; however, the Sloan Kettering Hospital study showed that multiply-transfused oncology patients had a significant rate of HTLV-1 seropositivity, suggesting that blood-borne HTLV contamination was a problem in clinical practice, even at the low seroprevalence rates noted above [118].

In the UK, HTLV-1 has been detected in approximately 5% of asymptomatic Caribbean immigrants [96, 119–121], including second generation children born in the UK, although HTLV-1 infection appears to be considerably less common in children born to infected mothers in the UK, than for children born in the Caribbean [121]. Between 4 and 5% of male homosexuals at risk for AIDS were HTLV-1 positive, and 6% of IV drug users were HTLV-2 infected [109]. One bizarre feature of the epidemiology of HTLV-1 to emerge recently is the occurrence of sporadic cases. In the UK, two clusters of family infections with HTLV-1 have been described in white caucasian men and their families who have never left the country, nor had exposure to any endemic area or contact [122, 123]. These small foci have been also reported from southern Italy and Sicily, France and from northern states of the USA [124–126]. As vertical transmission of this virus appears to be the major path of spread, and silent asymptomatic infection life-long is the rule, one can imagine that HTLV-1, introduced into a family by a traveller several generations previously, could remain in a family line for several generations [122].

(a) *HTLV-2: Special problems*

HTLV-2 was described first in 1982 from a patient with an unusual T cell variant of hairy cell leukaemia [9]; only one further isolate has ever been reported from this disease, and only five isolates are described in total [10]. There is complete serological overlap between these two viruses, but little cross-neutralization [19–21].

Competitive assays may distinguish HTLV-1 and -2, and data from surveys have shown that IV drug users have a 4–6% prevalence of HTLV-2 in both the UK and the USA [109, 120, 127]. The distribution of HTLV-2 around the world is not known, but no endemic group other than IV drug users has yet been described. As mentioned above, 21 of 23 New Orleans IV drug abusers, first identified as seropositive in an HTLV-1 test, are in fact HTLV-2-infected when analysed by more specific PCR analysis [110]. Prospective investigation of HTLV-2-infected subjects is now essential in order to investigate the natural history and pathogenicity of this virus.

(b) *Transmission of HTLV-1*

The exact mode(s) of transmission of HTLV-1 are unknown. The earliest data from Japan suggested that horizontal transmission occurred through sexual intercourse [128]. The increased prevalence of HTLV-1 in women in endemic areas has been explained by the greater relative efficiency of male-to-female transmission at intercourse, than vice versa. Sexual transmission is corroborated by the relatively higher rates of HTLV-1 in sexually active male homosexuals at risk for HIV [109, 120], and by the finding of an increased risk of HTLV-1 seropositivity in sexually promiscuous IV drug users matched for needle sharing [129]. However, a limited study of London prostitutes at risk for HTLV-1 through unprotected sexual intercourse with their West Indian boyfriends has shown no cases of HTLV-1 infection [130].

Mother-to-child transmission was reported *in utero* [131], and later via breast milk [132]. The latter route is favoured by the rabbit HTLV-1 model [133], where suckling transmits HTLV-1 efficiently, but the trans-placental route does not lead to infection in the offspring [134]. However, the placental anatomy of the rabbit does not allow direct comparison with man. The transmission of HTLV-1 in breast milk by the oral route to a common marmoset [135], the finding of HTLV-1 antigen in breast milk [136] and the higher prevalence of HTLV-1 infection in breast-fed children of infected mothers compared to bottle-fed [137, 138] all support post-natal transmission. However, caution must be exercised in the primal role of breast feeding, as the lower rate of HTLV-1 infection in children born to infected mothers in the UK, compared to those born to infected mothers in the Caribbean, suggests other factors relating to social deprivation may be in operation [113, 121].

Whole-blood transfusion has been repeatedly shown to be a significant route of transmission [139], and has been thought to account for up to 16% of all HTLV-1 infections in an endemic area in southern Japan [140]. The absence of HTLV-1 infection in haemophiliacs points to the cell-associated nature of HTLV-1 (see above), and the absence of the virus in plasma or plasma derivatives.

However, closer examination of the details of HTLV-1 distribution in the Caribbean poses questions as to this tidy view of the world. Miller [113] has shown that rates of HTLV-1 seropositivity rise with age, and that female infection is always more common than male; this has been confirmed by large serological studies [126, 141]. Infection was related to the quality of housing, with inferior social conditions producing significantly more infection; proximity to water and poor housing may implicate insect-borne transmission. Certainly, the distribution of HTLV-1 around the world is confined largely to the humid tropical belt, and within these areas HTLV-1 seropositivity is found predominantly in the coastal regions, where arthropod-borne diseases are more common [107]; however, populations tend to be concentrated in the littoral, and many infectious diseases are more common in this location. Intriguingly, many have noted that mother-to-child transmission of HTLV-1 is more common in children born to seropositive mothers in the Caribbean, than in children of seropositive Caribbean immigrant mothers, born in the UK [142]. Some factor applying to the tropics, and not to the UK, enhances transmission dramatically; this may be the social factors of poor housing and hygiene noted as independent risk factors in the Caribbean. Changes in these social factors may explain why the seroprevalence of HTLV-1 appears to be declining in endemic areas [143]. This effect has also been observed in southern Japan, where there is an increasing prevalence of HTLV-1 infection by age, without evidence from cohort studies that subjects seroconvert after the first year of life. The nature of the environmental changes leading to HTLV-1 decline in endemic populations are unknown.

Because of the observation that HTLV-2 is more common in drug abusers than homosexual men, one may suppose that transmission by blood is more efficient than by sex [120, 127]. No other transmission data on HTLV-2 are available.

7.7 CLINICAL ASPECTS OF DISEASES ASSOCIATED WITH HTLV INFECTION

7.7.1 Adult T cell leukaemia/lymphoma (ATL)

The first clinical description of ATL was published in 1977 by Uchiyama and Takatsuki [4]. It is a rapidly progressive acute leukaemia of T cell phenotype, which is unusual for the acute leukaemias (where over 95% are B cell or null cell phenotype). Patients present acutely, frequently have fever, generalized lymphadenopathy, hypercalcaemia and disseminated grade IV disease is often present on presentation; prognosis is poor [144]. The skin is often involved, with lesions varying from discrete or confluent nodules to plaques, patches and erythroderma, and this accounted for the initial confusion with Mycosis fungoides. The systemic complications include pleural effusion, aseptic meningitis and gastrointestinal tract involvement. The hypercalcaemia, which is invariably present, is associated with skeletal lesions, a high alkaline phosphatase and normal phosphate. Patients in the leukaemic phase are more susceptible to opportunist infections, and *Pneumocystis carinii* pneumonia, CMV, cryptococcosis and candidiasis have been described in association with HTLV-1 infection alone [145].

The leukaemic cells have a particular characteristic morphology, and biopsy of the lymph node, but rarely the skin lesions, also give diagnostic information. Peripheral blood lymphocytes from ATL patients will proliferate in cell culture, and it is possible to generate IL-2-independent cells. HTLV genome can be demonstrated in these cells, which are clonal. It is possible that pre-leukaemic stages of ATL exist [146], and asymptomatic carriers may have small numbers of abnormal circulating lymphocytes.

7.7.2 Tropical spastic paraparesis (TSP)

While studying the seroprevalence of HTLV-1 on Martinique, Gessain observed that there was a strong association between HTLV-1 infection and tropical spastic paraparesis [147], a syndrome first described by Montgomery and Cruikshank in 1964 [148]. Further studies by Newton on Caribbean immigrants in London, Rodgers-Johnson *et al.* in the Caribbean and others have confirmed this epidemiological association [149, 150]. Moreover, Japanese investigators have noted a syndrome termed the HTLV-associated myelopathy (HAM), which is clinically indistinguishable from TSP [151]. HAM cases have been observed following transfusion-associated HTLV-1 infection in Japan, as well as with perinatally or horizontally acquired infection [152]. HTLV-1-associated TSP has now also been described from temperate zones, including Santiago in Chile [153] and southern Italy [154], and so a change of nomenclature is clearly desirable.

The virological association of TSP/HAM with HTLV-1 is now far from circumstantial. In addition to the serological association of HTLV-1 antibodies to TSP, which approaches 100% correlation in some series [149], HTLV-1 virus has been isolated from the CSF of these patients [100]. CSF isolates from TSP have recently been shown to be closely related by nucleotide sequence and restriction enzyme polymorphism to the virus found in lymphocytes in ATL cases [101, 102, 155]. There is intra-thecal synthesis of anti-HTLV-1 IgG in the CSF [156], and it is possible to find abnormal, pleomorphic lymphocytes in the peripheral blood of TSP/HAM patients which resemble the abnormal lymphocytes seen in the pre-leukaemic stage of ATL [157, 158]. One case has been reported of an HTLV-1 seropositive patient with both TSP and ATL [159]. The pathogenesis of HTLV in the CNS is unknown; there are very high antibody titres to HTLV-1 in the CSF and serum of TSP patients compared to ATL patients, and this may possibly reflect an immunological basis to TSP, whereby cross-reacting antibodies between HTLV-1 and a host protein such as myelin basic protein leads to "autoimmune" damage to the CNS [157]; an immunological association involving cytotoxic T cells is also a much favoured hypothesis, for which no data currently exist.

The clinical features of TSP/HAM are distinctive, and quite separate from the more common idiopathic demyelinating disease, multiple sclerosis (MS). The disease presents initially between the ages of 20 and 50 years, with lumbar back pain radiating down the legs as the commonest presenting symptom. The criteria for diagnosis are:

In patients with no childhood history of weakness, two of the following must be present within 2 years of onset:

Low back and leg pain;
Urinary frequency, nocturia and/or retention of urine;
Symmetrical weakness within 6 months;
Dysaesthesiae/anaesthesiae of the lower limbs.

Clinical examination should show spasticity of the lower limbs, with increased patellar reflexes, no sensory level and no pupillary changes; upper limb signs may occur later in the disease. There must be no history of relapse or remission, which is the characteristic of the MS presentation in the older patient, where lower limb long tract signs may predominate.

CSF examination characteristically shows a lymphocytic pleocytosis with raised protein levels, normal glucose and oligoclonal bands. In the tropics, the major differential diagnoses are: (1) meningovascular syphilis; (2) syringomyelia; (3) spinal schistosomiasis; (4) transverse myelitis. In the West, the major differential diagnosis is MS, and so the history of chronic progression against relapse and remission are of some importance. The neurophysiological parameters of MS may also be found to be abnormal in TSP, and the visual and auditory evoked potentials may be identical. Magnetic resonance imaging (MRI) may show the extensive plaques associated with MS which are *not* a feature of TSP, but CT scanning may be less useful [148, 160]. MRI abnormalities may also be seen in the brain of asymptomatic HTLV-1 carriers [161]. Pathologically, TSP shows a lymphocytic perivascular cuffing in the spinal cord, and meningeal inflammation.

It is clear from the above discussion that the finding of a virus associated with an MS-like disease is of interest to the possible aetiology of MS itself. There have been reports of a serological association between antibodies to HTLV-1 p24 and MS, and subsequently the amplification of the HTLV-1 genome from a HTLV-1 seronegative patient with MS by the PCR technique [162, 163]. However, the serological association between HTLV-1 and MS has not been confirmed [164, 165], and anxieties concerning PCR contamination mean that this report is both unconfirmed and to be treated with caution at this time [166, 167]. However, this is a rapidly evolving field, and the discovery of a retrovirus associated with demyelination is still of considerable importance.

7.7.3   Other disease associations of HTLV

As risk groups for HTLV and HIV are shared, it is not surprising that doubly-infected subjects have been found. Studies in Trinidad have suggested that doubly-infected patients, who have antibodies to both HTLV-1 and to HIV-1, have a higher rate of conversion to AIDS after infection by HIV [168]. This requires further study. Two reports of dual infection leading to a CD8+ T cell lympho-proliferative disease have been published [169, 170]. HTLV-1 associated polymyositis has recently been reported in a subject co-infected with HIV-1 [171]; this study suggested direct HTLV-1 infection of muscle tissue. Larger studies from an endemic area in the Caribbean suggest that 11/13 (85%) of subjects with idiopathic adult polymyositis have antibodies to HTLV-1 [172]. These cases all demonstrate a marked lymphocytic infiltrate into the muscle tissue.

The importance of continued vigilance for the development of new clinical syndromes in dual infection must be stressed. A recent report suggests that ATL patients have a high rate of multiple primary malignancies [173], and further oncological sequelae of HTLV infection need to be sought. The prevalence of immunological abnormality in otherwise asymptomatic HTLV-1 carriers is unknown; a report from Japan shows suppression of tuberculin delayed type hypersensitivity reactivity (anergy) in healthy HTLV-1-infected subjects compared to geographically and age-matched controls [174].

Other, rare and largely unconfirmed clinical associations of HTLV-1 include Sjögren's syndrome [175], T cell alveolitis [176] and large granular lymphocyte proliferative disorders [177], and a case report of HTLV-1-associated chronic inflammatory arthropathy [178]. Reports of the association of HTLV-1 with MS and with mycosis fungoides must be treated with caution at this time (see above).

7.7.4 Counselling the HTLV-infected patient

The natural history of HTLV-1 suggests that there is a 4.5% cumulative life-time risk of ATL development for males, and a 2.6% life-time risk of ATL in an infected female [116]. Similar figures, though without the male bias, of a cumulative life-time risk of ATL of 4.0–4.2% in those infected by HTLV-1 before the age of 20 years have been found by computer modelling [179]. The life-time chance of TSP/HAM developing is not yet known, but may be slightly higher. It is not yet known whether there are any other consequences of infection, nor whether HTLV-2 infection has these or different sequelae.

HTLV-infected subjects should never give blood, bone marrow, breast milk, semen or any organ, and should not carry organ donor cards.

It is extremely difficult to explain the concept of a persistent leukaemia virus infection, which may be silent life-long, yet is transmissable to partners and children. Counselling asymptomatic carriers is almost always extremely time-consuming, and the uncertainty over clinical outcome can be frustrating for even the most intelligent and informed subject. The practical difficulties in what to tell the patient imply that screening should be undertaken only in full realization of the onus placed on subjects identified as harbouring HTLV-1. The difficulties in testing for HTLV-2 are even more problematic, as there is still uncertainty as to whether this is a pathogenic virus. Physicians testing for these viruses must be prepared to accept the consequences of counselling, and obtaining patients' consent to testing should be considered mandatory.

REFERENCES

1. Gallo, R.C. (1986). HTLV-1 — The first human retrovirus. *Scient. Am.* (December), 78–88.
2. Weiss, R.A. (1985). Human T-cell retroviruses. In *RNA Tumor Viruses*, 2nd edn (Weiss, R., Teich, N., Varmus, H. and Coffin, J., eds), pp. 405–485. Cold Spring Harbor Laboratory, Cold Spring Harbor.
3. Poiecz, B., Ruscetti, F., Gazdar, A. *et al.* (1980). Detection and isolation of type C retrovirus particles from fresh and cultured lymphocytes of a patient with cutaneous T-cell lymphoma. *Proc. Natl Acad. Sci. USA* **77**, 7415–7419.
4. Uchiyama, T., Yodoi, J., Sagawa, K., Takatsuki, K. and Uchino, H. (1977).

Adult T-cell leukaemia; clinical and haematological features of 16 cases. *Blood* **50**, 481–492.

5. Hinuma, Y., Nagata, K., Hanaoka, M. *et al.* (1981). Adult T-cell leukaemia: Antigen in an ATL cell line and detection of antibodies to the antigen in human sera. *Proc. Natl Acad. Sci. USA* **78**, 6476–6480.

6. Miyoshi, I., Kubonishi, I., Yoshimoto, S. *et al.* (1981). Type C retrovirus in a cord blood T-cell line derived by co-cultivating normal human leukaemic T-cells. *Nature, Lond.* **294**, 770–771.

7. Hinuma, Y., Komoda, H., Chosa, T. *et al.* (1982). Antibody to adult T-cell leukaemia virus associated antigen (ATLA) in sera from patients with ATL and controls in Japan: A nationwide sero-epidemiologic study. *Int. J. Cancer* **29**, 631–635.

8. Watanabe, T., Seiki, M. and Yoshida, M. (1984). HTLV Type I (US isolate) and ATLV (Japanese isolate) are the same species of human retrovirus. *Virology* **133**, 238–241.

9. Kalyanaraman, V., Sarngadharan, M., Robert-Guroff, M. *et al.* (1982). A new subtype of human T-cell leukaemia virus (HTLV-2) associated with a T-cell variant of hairy cell leukaemia. *Science* **218**, 571–573.

10. Rosenblatt, J., Golde, D., Wachsman, W. *et al.* (1986). A second isolate of HTLV-2 associated with atypical hairy cell leukaemia. *New Engl. J. Med.* **315**, 372–377.

11. Miyoshi, I., Fujishita, M., Taguchi, H. *et al.* (1983). Natural infection in non-human primates with adult T-cell leukaemia virus or a closely related agent. *Int. J. Cancer* **32**, 333–336.

12. Hunsmann, G., Schneider, J., Schmitt, J. and Yamamoto, N. (1983). Detection of serum antibodies to adult T-cell leukaemia virus in non-human primates and in people from Africa. *Int. J. Cancer* **32**, 329–332.

13. Tsujimoto, H., Komuro, A., Iijima, K., Miyamoto, J., Ishikawa, K. and Hayami, M. (1985). Isolation of simian retroviruses closely related to human T-cell leukemia virus by establishment of lymphoid cell lines from various non-human primates. *Int. J. Cancer* **35**, 377–384.

14. Clapham, P., Nagy, K., Cheingsong-Popov, R., Exley, M. and Weiss, R.A. (1983). Productive infection and cell-free transmission of human T-cell leukemia virus in a nonlymphoid cell line. *Science* **222**, 1125–1127.

15. Ho, D.D., Rota, T.R. and Hirsch, M.S. (1984). Infection of human endothelial cells by human T-lymphotropic virus type 1. *Proc. Natl Acad. Sci. USA* **81**, 7588–7590.

16. Hoxie, J.A., Matthews, D.M. and Cines, D.B. (1984). Infection of human endothelial cells by human T-cell leukemia virus type 1. *Proc. Natl Acad. Sci. USA* **81**, 7591–7595.

17. Nagy, K., Clapham, P., Cheingsong-Popov, R. and Weiss, R.A. (1983). Human T-cell leukaemia virus type I: Induction of syncytia and inhibition by patients' sera. *Int. J. Cancer* **32**, 321–328.

18. Hoshino, H., Shimoyama, M., Miwa, M. and Sugimara, T. (1983). Detection of lymphocytes producing a human retrovirus associated with adult T-cell leukemia by syncytia induction assay. *Proc. Natl Acad. Sci. USA* **80**, 7337–7341.

19. Clapham, P.R., Nagy, K. and Weiss, R.A. (1984). Pseudotypes of human T-cell leukemia virus types 1 and 2: Neutralization by patients' sera. *Proc. Natl Acad. Sci. USA* **81**, 2886–2889.

20. Weiss, R.A., Clapham, P., Nagy, K. and Hoshino, H. (1985). Envelope properties of human T-cell leukemia viruses. *Curr. Topics Microbiol. Immunol.* **115**, 235–246.

21. Hoshino, H., Clapham, P.R., Weiss, R.A., Miyoshi, I., Yoshida, M. and Miwa, M. (1985). Human T-cell leukemia virus type I: pseudotype neutralisation of Japanese and American isolates with human and rabbit sera. *Int. J. Cancer* **36**, 671–675.

22. Sommerfelt, M.A., Williams, B.P., Clapham, P.R., Solomon, E., Goodfellow, P.N. and Weiss, R.A. (1988). Human T cell leukemia viruses use a receptor determined by human chromosome 17. *Science* **242**, 1557–1559.

23. Seiki, M., Hattori, S., Hirayama, Y. and Yoshida, M. (1983). Human adult T-cell leukemia virus: Complete nucleotide sequence of the provirus genome integrated in leukemia cell DNA. *Proc. Natl Acad. Sci. USA* **80**, 3618–3622.

24. Malik, K.T.A., Even, J. and Karpas, A. (1988). Molecular cloning and complete nucleotide sequence of an adult T cell leukaemia virus/human T cell leukaemia virus type 1 (ATLV/HTLV-1) isolate of Caribbean origin: Relationship to other members of the ATLV/HTLV-1 subgroup. *J. Gen. Virol.* **69**, 1695–1710.

25. Sagata, N., Yasunaga, T., Tsuzuku-Kawamura, J., Ohishi, K., Ogawa, Y. and Ikawa, Y. (1985). Complete nucleotide sequence of the genome of bovine leukemia virus: Its evolutionary relationship to other retroviruses. *Proc. Natl Acad. Sci. USA* **82**, 677–681.

26. Watanabe, T., Seiki, M., Tsujimoto, H., Miyoshi, I., Hayami, M. and Yoshida, M. (1985). Sequence homology of the simian retrovirus genome with human T-cell leukemia virus type I. *Virology* **144**, 59–65.

27. Ratner, L., Haseltine, W., Patarca, R. *et al.* (1985). Complete nucleotide sequence of the AIDS-virus, HTLV-III. *Nature, Lond.* **313**, 277–284.

28. Chakrabarti, L., Guyader, M., Alizon, M. *et al.* (1987). Sequence of Simian immunodeficiency virus from macaque and its relationship to other human and Simian retroviruses. *Nature, Lond.* **328**, 543–547.

29. Paskalis, H., Felber, B.K. and Pavlakis, G.N. (1986). *Cis*-acting sequences responsible for the transcriptional activation of human T-cell leukaemia virus type I constitute a conditional enhancer. *Proc. Natl Acad. Sci. USA* **83**, 6558–6562.

30. Shimotohno, K., Takano, M., Teruuchi, T. and Miwa, M. (1986). Requirement of multiple copies of a 21-nucleotide sequence in the U3 region of human T-cell leukaemia virus type I and type II long terminal repeats for transacting activation of transcription. *Proc. Natl Acad. Sci. USA* **83**, 8112–8116.

31. Tsukada, T., Fink, J.S., Mandel, G. and Goodman, R.H. (1987). Identification of a region in the human vasoactive intestinal polypeptide gene responsible for regulation by cyclic AMP. *J. Biol. Chem.* **262**, 8743–8747.

32. Jeang, K.-T., Boros, I., Brady, J., Radonovich, M. and Khoury, G. (1988). Characterization of cellular factors that interact with the human T-cell leukemia virus type I p40^x responsive 21-base-pair sequence. *J. Virol.* **62**, 4499–4509.

33. Nerenberg, M., Hinrichs, S.H., Reynolds, R.K., Khoury, G. and Jay, G.

(1987). The *tat* gene of human T-lymphotropic virus type 1 induces mesenchymal tumors in transgenic mice. *Science* **237**, 1324–1329.

34. Furuta, Y., Aizawa, S., Suda, Y. *et al.* (1989). Thymic atrophy characteristic in transgenic mice that harbour pX genes of human T-cell leukemia virus type I. *J. Virol.* **63**, 3185–3189.

35. Hinrichs, S.H., Nerenberg, M., Reynolds, R.K., Khoury, G. and Jay, G. (1987). A transgenic mouse model for human neurofibromatosis. *Science* **237**, 1340–1343.

36. Guyader, M., Emerman, M., Sonigo, P., Clavel, F., Montagnier, L. and Alizon, M. (1987). Genome organization and transactivation of the human immunodeficiency virus type 2. *Nature, Lond.* **326**, 662–669.

37. Seiki, M., Hikikoshi, A., Taniguchi, T. and Yoshida, M. (1985). Expression of the pX gene of HTLV-1: General splicing mechanism in the HTLV family. *Science* **228**, 1532–1534.

38. Hattori, S., Kiyokawa, T., Imagawa, K.T. *et al.* (1984). Identification of *gag* and *env* gene products of human T-cell leukaemia virus (HTLV). *Virology* **136**, 338–347.

39. Copeland, T.D., Oroszlan, S., Kalyanaraman, V.S., Sarngadharan, M.G. and Gallo, R.C. (1983). Complete amino acid sequence of human T-cell leukemia virus structural protein p15. *FEBS Lett.* **162**, 390–395.

40. Oroszlan, S., Sarujadharan, M.G., Copeland, T.D., Kalyanaran, V.S., Gilden, R.V. and Gallo, R.C. (1982). Primary structure analysis of the major internal protein p24 of human type C T-cell leukemia virus. *Proc. Natl Acad. Sci. USA* **79**, 1291–1294.

41. Nam, S.H., Kidokoro, M., Shida, H. and Hatanaka, M. (1988). Processing of *gag* precursor polyprotein of human T-cell leukemia virus type I by virus-encoded protease. *J. Virol.* **62**, 3718–3728.

42. Rho, H.M., Poiesz, B.J., Ruscetti, F.W. and Gallo, R.C. (1981). Characterization of the reverse transcriptase from a new retrovirus (HTLV) produced by a human cutaneous T-cell lymphoma cell line. *Virology* **112**, 355–360.

43. Kiokawa, T., Yoshikura, H., Hattori, S., Seiki, M. and Yoshida, M. (1984). Envelope proteins of human T-cell leukaemia virus: Expression in *Escherichia coli* and its application to studies of *env* function. *Proc. Natl Acad. Sci. USA* **81**, 6202–6206.

44. Nakamura, H., Hayami, M., Ohta, Y. *et al.* (1987). Protection of cynomolgus monkeys against infection by human T-cell leukemia virus type I by immunization with viral *env* gene products produced in *Escherichia coli. Int. J. Cancer* **40**, 403–407.

45. Shida, Y., Tochikura, T., Sato, T. *et al.* (1987). Effect of the recombinant vaccinia viruses that express HTLV-I envelope gene on HTLV-I infection. *EMBO J.* **6**, 3379–3384.

46. Palker, T.J., Tanner, M.E., Scearce, R.M., Streilein, R.D., Clark, M.E. and Haynes, B.F. (1989). Mapping of immunogenic regions of human T cell leukemia virus type I (HTLV-I) gp46 and gp21 envelope glycoproteins with *env*-encoded synthetic peptides and a monoclonal antibody to gp46. *J. Immunol.* **142**, 971–978.

47. Burny, A., Bruck, C., Cleuter, Y. *et al.* (1985). Bovine leukemia virus, a distinguished member of the human T-lymphotropic virus family. In *Retroviruses in Human Lymphoma/Leukemia* (M. Miwa *et al.*, eds),

pp. 219–227. Tokyo Science Press, Tokyo.

48. Portetelle, D., Dandoy, C., Burny, A. *et al.* (1989). Synthetic peptides approach to identification of epitopes on Bovine Leukemia Virus envelope glycoprotein gp51. *Virology* **169**, 34–41.

49. Snyderman, R. and Cianciolo, G.J. (1984). Immunosuppressive activity of the retroviral envelope protein P15E and its possible relationship to neoplasia. *Immunol. Today* **5**, 240–244.

50. Cianciolo, G.J., Copeland, T.D., Oroszlan, S. and Snyderman, R. (1985). Inhibition of lymphocyte proliferation by a synthetic peptide homologous to retroviral envelope proteins. *Science* **230**, 453–455.

51. Nagashima, K., Yoshida, M. and Seiki, M. (1986). A single species of pX mRNA of human T-cell leukemia virus type I encodes *trans*-activator p40^x and two other phosphoroproteins. *J. Virol.* **60**, 394–399.

52. Kiyokawa, T., Seiki, M., Iwashita, S., Imagawa, K., Shimizu, F. and Yoshida, M. (1985). p27x-III and p21x-III, proteins encoded by the pX sequence of human T-cell leukemia virus type I. *Proc. Natl Acad. Sci. USA* **82**, 8359–8363.

53. Inoue, J.-I., Yoshida, M. and Seiki, M. (1987). Transcriptional (p40x) and post-transcriptional (p27x-III) regulators are required for the expression and replication of human T-cell leukemia virus type I genes. *Proc. Natl Acad. Sci. USA* **84**, 3653–3657.

54. Sodroski, J., Rosen, C., Goh, W.C. and Haseltine, W. (1985). A transcriptional activator protein encoded by the x-*lor* region of the human T-cell leukemia virus. *Science* **228**, 1430–1434.

55. Slamon, D.J., Shimotohno, K., Cline, M.J., Golde, D.W. and Chen, I.S.Y. (1984). Identification of the putative transforming proteins of the human T-cell leukemia viruses HTLV-I and HTLV-II. *Science* **226**, 61–64.

56. Lee, T.H., Coligan, J.E., Sodroski, J.G. *et al.* (1984). Antigens encoded by the 3′-terminal region of human T-cell leukemia virus: Evidence for a functional gene. *Science* **226**, 57–61.

57. Seiki, M., Inoue, J., Takeda, T. and Yoshida, M. (1986). Direct evidence that p40x of human T-cell leukemia virus type I is a *trans*-acting transcriptional activator. *EMBO J.* **5**, 561–565.

58. Sodroski, J.G., Rosen, C.A. and Haseltine, W.A. (1984). *Trans*-acting transcriptional activation of the long terminal repeat of human T lymphotropic viruses in infected cells. *Science* **225**, 381–385.

59. Fujisawa, J., Seiki, M., Kiyokawa, T. and Yoshida, M. (1985). Functional activation of the long terminal repeat of human T-cell leukemia virus type I by a *trans*-acting factor. *Proc. Natl Acad. Sci. USA* **82**, 2277–2281.

60. Felber, B.K., Paskalis, H., Kleinman-Ewing, C., Wong-Staal, F. and Pavlakis, G.N. (1985). The pX protein of HTLV-I is a transcriptional activator of its own long terminal repeats. *Science* **229**, 675–679.

61. Siekevitz, M., Feinberg, M.B., Holbrook, N., Wong-Staal, F. and Greene, W.C. (1987). Activation of interleukin 2 and interleukin 2 receptor (Tac) promoter expression by the trans-activator (*tat*) gene product of human T-cell leukemia virus, type I. *Proc. Natl Acad. Sci. USA* **84**, 5389–5393.

62. Greene, W.C., Leonard, W.J., Wano, Y. *et al.* (1986). *Trans*-activator gene of HTLV-II induces IL-2 receptor and IL-2 cellular gene expression. *Science* **232**, 877–880.

63. Inoue, J., Seiki, M., Taniguchi, T., Tsuru, S. and Yoshida, M. (1986).

Induction of interleukin 2 receptor gene expression by p40x encoded by human T-cell leukemia virus type 1. *EMBO J.* **5**, 2883–2888.

64. Maruyama, M., Shibuya, H., Harada, H. *et al.* (1987). Evidence for aberrant activation of the interleukin-2 autocrine loop by HTLV-1 encoded p40x and T3/Ti complex triggering. *Cell* **48**, 343–350.

65. Cross, S.L., Feinberg, M.B., Wolf, J.B., Holbrook, N.J., Wong-Staal, F. and Leonard, W.J. (1987). Regulation of the human interleukin-2 receptor α chain promotor: Activation of a nonfunctional promoter by the transactivator gene of HTLV-1. *Cell* **49**, 47–56.

66. Arai, N., Nomura, D., Villaret, D. *et al.* (1989). Complete nucleotide sequence of the chromosomal gene for human IL-4 and its expression. *J. Immunol.* **142**, 274–282.

67. Miyatake, S., Seiki, M., DeWaal Malefijt, R. *et al.* (1988). Activation of T cell-derived lymphokine genes in T cells and fibroblasts: effects of human T cell leukemia virus type I p40x protein and bovine papilloma virus encoded E2 protein. *Nucleic Acids Res.* **16**, 6547–6566.

68. Fujii, M., Sassone-Corsi, P. and Verma, I.M. (1988). C-*fos* promoter trans-activation by the tax1 protein of human T-cell leukemia virus type I. *Proc. Natl Acad. Sci. USA* **85**, 8526–8530.

69. Wano, Y., Feinberg, M., Hosking, J.B., Bogerd, H. and Greene, W.C. (1988). Stable expression of the *tax* gene of type I human T-cell leukemia virus in human T cell activates specific cellular genes involved in growth. *Proc. Natl Acad. Sci. USA* **85**, 9733–9737.

70. Slamon, D.J., Boyle, W.J., Keith, D.E., Press, M.F., Golde, D.W. and Souza, L.M. (1988). Subnuclear localization of the *trans*-activating protein of human T-cell leukemia virus Type I. *J. Virol.* **62**, 680–686.

71. Brady, J., Jeang, K.T., Duvall, J. and Khoury, G. (1987). Identification of p40[x]-responsive regulatory sequences within the human T-cell leukemia virus Type I long terminal repeat. *J. Virol.* **61**, 2175–2181.

72. Fujisawa, J., Seiki, M., Sato, M. and Yoshida, M. (1986). A transcriptional enhancer sequence of HTLV-1 is responsible for transactivation mediated by p40[x] of HTLV-I. *EMBO J.* **5**, 713–718.

73. Ballard, D.W., Böhnlein, E., Lowenthal, J.W., Wano, Y., Franza, B.R. and Greene, W.C. (1988). HTLV-I tax induces cellular proteins that activate the kB element in the IL-2 α gene. *Science* **241**, 1652–1655.

74. Leung, K. and Nabel, G.J. (1988). HTLV-1 transactivator induces interleukin-2 receptor expression through an NF-kB-like factor. *Nature, Lond.* **333**, 776–778.

75. Kai, C., Okada, N. and Okada, H. (1988). Expression of CR2 (C3d receptor) on the cell membranes of adult T cell leukemia. *Jpn. J. Cancer Res.* **79**, 805–808.

76. Schulz, T.F., Petzer, A., Stauder, R., Eigentler, A. and Dierich, M.P. (1986). Expression of CR2 (C3d/EBV-receptor) on HTLV-1 transformed human T-cells. *Abstracts 6th International Congress on Immunology,* Toronto (Abstract 2.51.14, pp. 188, 356).

77. Pantazis, P., Sariban, E., Bohan, C.A., Antoniades, H.N. and Kalyanaraman, V.S. (1987). Synthesis of PDGF by cultured human T cells transformed with HTLV-I and II. *Oncogene* **1**, 285–289.

78. Kingston, R.E., Baldwin, A.S. and Sharp, P.A. (1985). Transcription control by oncogenes. *Cell* **41**, 3–5.

79. Green, M.R. (1989). When the products of oncogenes and anti-oncogenes meet. *Cell* **56**, 1–3.
80. Dingwall, C., Ernberg, I., Heaphey, S., Skinner, M., Gait, M. and Karn, J. (1989). Binding of the HIV-1 tat protein to tar sequences *in vitro*. *Vth International Conference on AIDS*, Montreal, June 1989 (Abstract T.C.O. 29, p. 520).
81. Rappaport, J., Josephs, S., Klotman, M. *et al.* (1989). Binding of HIV-1 tat to the 5' region of mRNA. *Vth International Conference on AIDS*, Montreal, June 1989 (Abstract T.C.O. 31, p. 520).
82. Seiki, M., Inoue, J., Hidaka, M. and Yoshida, M. (1988). Two *cis*-acting elements responsible for posttranscriptional *trans*-regulation of gene expression of human T-cell leukemia virus type I. *Proc. Natl Acad. Sci. USA* **85**, 7124–7128.
83. Hidaka, M., Inoue, J., Yoshida, M. and Seiki, M. (1988). Posttranscriptional regulator (*rex*) of HTLV-1 initiates expression of viral structural proteins but suppresses expression of regulatory proteins. *EMBO J.* **7**, 519–523.
84. Rimsky, L., Hauber, J., Dukovich, M. *et al.* (1988). Functional replacement of the HIV-1 *rev* protein by the HTLV-1 *rex* protein. *Nature, Lond.* **335**, 738–740.
85. Malim, M.H., Hauber, J., Le, S.-Y., Maizel, J.V. and Cullen, B.R. (1989). The HIV-1 *rev trans*-activator acts through a structured target sequence to activate nuclear export of unspliced viral mRNA. *Nature, Lond.* **338**, 254–257.
86. Markham, P.D., Salahuddin, S.Z., Kalyanaraman, V.S., Popovic, M., Sarin, P. and Gallo, R.C. (1983). Infection and transformation of fresh human umbilical cord blood cells by multiple sources of human T-cell leukemia-lymphoma virus (HTLV). *Int. J. Cancer* **31**, 413–420.
87. Faller, D.V., Crimmins, M.A.V. and Mentzer, S.J. (1988). Human T-cell leukemia virus type I infection of CD4+ or CD8+ cytotoxic T-cell clones results in immortalization with retention of antigen specificity. *J. Virol.* **62**, 2942–2950.
88. Gazzolo, L. and Dodon, M.D. (1987). Direct activation of resting T lymphocytes by human T-lymphotropic virus type I. *Nature, Lond.* **326**, 714–717.
89. Melchers, F., Erdei, A., Schulz, T.F. and Dierich, M.P. (1985). Growth control of activated, synchronized murine B cells by the C3d fragment of human complement. *Nature, Lond.* **317**, 264–267.
90. Nemerow, G.R., McNaughton, M.E. and Cooper, N.R. (1985). Binding of monoclonal antibody to the Epstein-Barr virus (EBV)/CR2 receptor induces activation and differentiation of human B-lymphocytes. *J. Immunol.* **135**, 3068–3072.
91. Petzer, A.L., Schulz, T.F., Stauder, R., Eigentler, A., Myones, B.L. and Dierich, M.P. (1988). Structural and functional analysis of CR2/EBV receptor by means of monoclonal antibodies and limited tryptic digestion. *Immunology* **63**, 47–53.
92. Seiki, M., Eddy, R., Shows, T.B. and Yoshida, M. (1984). Nonspecific integration of the HTLV provirus genome into adult T-cell leukaemia cells. *Nature, Lond.* **309**, 640–642.
93. Hiramatsu, K. and Yoshikura, H. (1986). Frequent partial deletion of

human adult T-cell leukemia virus type I provirus in experimental transmission: Pattern and possible implication. *J. Virol.* **58**, 508–512.

94. Tsudo, M., Uchiyama, T., Uchino, H. and Yodoi, J. (1983). Failure of regulation of *tac* antigen/TCGF receptor on adult T-cell leukemia cells by anti-*tac* monoclonal antibody. *Blood* **61**, 1014–1016.

95. Franchini, G., Wong-Staal, F. and Gallo, R.C. (1984). Human T-cell leukemia virus (HTLV-1) transcripts in fresh and cultured cells of patients with adult T-cell leukemia. *Proc. Natl Acad. Sci. USA* **81**, 6207–6211.

96. Matutes, E., Dalgleish, A.G., Weiss, R.A., Joseph, A.P. and Catovsky, D. (1986). Studies in healthy human T-cell-leukemia lymphoma virus (HTLV-I) carriers from the Caribbean. *Int. J. Cancer* **38**, 41–45.

97. Miyamoto, K., Tomita, N., Ishii, A. *et al.* (1984). Chromosomal abnormalities of leukemia cells in adult patients with T-cell leukemia. *J. Natl Cancer Inst.* **73**, 353–359.

98. Miyamoto, K., Tomita, N., Ishii, A. *et al.* (1987). Specific abnormalities of chromosome 14 in patients with acute type of adult T-cell leukemia/lymphoma. *Int. J. Cancer* **40**, 461–468.

99. Lenoir, G.M. and Bornkamm, G.W. (1987). Burkitt's lymphoma, a human cancer model for the study of the multistep development of cancer: proposal for a new scenario. *Adv. Viral Oncol.* **7**, 173–206.

100. Gessain, A., Saal, F., Morozov, V. *et al.* (1989). Characterization of HTLV-1 isolates and T lymphoid cell lines derives from French West Indian patients with tropical spastic paraparesis. *Int. J. Cancer* **43**, 327–333.

101. Bangham, C.R.M., Daenke, S., Phillips, R.E., Cruickshank, J.K. and Bell, J.I. (1988), Enzymatic amplification of exogenous and endogenous retroviral sequences from DNA of patients with tropical spastic paraparesis. *EMBO J.* **7**, 4179–4184.

102. Kwok, S., Kellogg, D., Ehrlich, G., Poiesz, B., Bhagavati, S. and Sninsky, J.J. (1988). Characterization of a sequence of human T-cell leukemia virus type I from a patient with chronic progressive myelopathy. *J. Infect. Dis.* **158**, 1193–1197.

103. Schupbach, J., Kalyanaraman, V., Sarngadharan, M. *et al.* (1983). Antibodies against three structural proteins of the human type C retrovirus, HTLV, in Japanese adult T-cell leukaemia patients, healthy family members and unrelated normals. *Int. J. Cancer* **32**, 583–590.

104. Yamamoto, N. and Hinuma, Y. (1982). Antigens in an adult T-cell leukaemia virus producer cell line: reactivity with human serum antibodies. *Int. J. Cancer* **30**, 289–293.

105. Slamon, D., Shimotohno, K., Cline, M., Golde, D. and Chen, I.S. (1984). Identification of the putative transforming protein of HTLV-1 and HTLV-2. *Science* **226**, 61–65.

106. Ehrlich, G.D., Glaser, J.B., Abbott, M.A. *et al.* (1989). Detection of anti-HTLV-I *tax* antibodies in HTLV-I enzyme linked immunosorbent assay negative individuals. *Blood* **74**, 1066–1072.

107. Weber, J., Banatvala, N., Clayden, S. *et al.* (1989). HTLV-1 infection in Papua New Guinea; evidence for serological false positivity. *J. Infect. Dis.* **159**, 1025–1028.

108. Mortimer, P., Parry, J. and Mortimer, J.Y. (1985). Which anti-HTLV-III/LAV assays for screening and confirmatory testing. *Lancet* **ii**, 873–876.

109. Tedder, R.S., Shanson, D.C., Jeffries, D. *et al.* (1984). Low prevalence in the UK of HTLV-1 and HTLV-III infection in subjects with AIDS, lymphadenopathy syndrome and at risk of AIDS. *Lancet* **ii**, 125–127.

110. Lee, H., Swanson, P., Shorty, V.S., Zack, J.A., Rosenblatt, J.D. and Chen, I.S. (1989). High rate of HTLV-2 infection in seropositive IV drug users in New Orleans. *Science* **244**, 471–475.

111. Duggan, D.B., Ehrlich, G.D., Davey, F.P. *et al.* (1988). HTLV-I induced lymphoma mimicking Hodgkin's disease. Diagnosis by polymerase chain reaction amplification of specific HTLV-I sequences in tumor DNA. *Blood* **71**, 1027–1032.

112. Blattner, W., Kalyanaraman, V., Robert-Guroff, M. *et al.* (1982). The human C-type retrovirus, HTLV, in blacks from the Caribbean and their relationship to adult T-cell leukaemia/lymphoma. *Int. J. Cancer* **30**, 257–264.

113. Miller, G., Pegram, S., Kirkwood, B. *et al.* (1986). Ethnic composition, age and sex together with location and standard of housing as determinants of HTLV-1 infection in an urban Trinidadian community. *Int. J. Cancer* **38**, 801–808.

114. Riedel, D., Evans, A.S., Saxinger, S. and Blattner, W. (1989). A historical study of HTLV-1 transmission in Barbados. *J. Infect. Dis.* **159**, 603–609.

115. Ueda, K., Kusuhara, K. and Tokugawa, K. (1988). Transmission of HTLV-1. *Lancet* **i**, 1163–1164.

116. Tokudome, S., Tokunaga, O., Shiramoto, S. *et al.* (1989). Incidence of adult T-cell leukaemia/lymphoma among human T-lymphotropic virus type 1 carriers in Japan. *Cancer Res.* **49**, 226–228.

117. Williams, A., Fang, C., Slamon, D. *et al.* (1988). Sero-prevalence and epidemiologic correlates of HTLV-1 infection in US blood donors. *Science* **240**, 643–646.

118. Minamoto, G., Gold, J., Scheinberg, D. *et al.* (1988). Infection with human T-cell leukaemia virus type 1 in patients with leukaemia. *New Engl. J. Med.* **318**, 219–222.

119. Catovsky, D., Greaves, M.F., Rose, M., Galton, D.A., Goolden, A. *et al.* (1982). Adult T-cell lymphoma/leukaemia in blacks from the West Indies. *Lancet* **i**, 639–643.

120. Robert-Guroff, M., Blayney, D., Safai, B. *et al.* (1984). HTLV-1 specific antibodies in AIDS patients and others at risk. *Lancet* **ii**, 128–130.

121. Tosswill, J., Peckham, C., Mortimer, P. and Weber, J. (1990). Epidemiology of HTLV-1 in an inner London ante-natal clinic. *Br. Med. J.* (in press).

122. Wyld, P., Tosswill, J., Mortimer, P. and Weber, J. (1990). HTLV-1 in an atypical host in the UK. *Br. J. Haematol.* (in press).

123. Cunningham, D., Gilchrist, N., Jack, A. *et al.* (1985). T-lymphoma associated with HTLV-1 outside the Caribbean and Japan. *Lancet* **ii**, 337–338.

124. Manzari, V., Gradilone, A., Barillari, G. *et al.* (1985). HTLV-1 is endemic in Southern Italy: detection of the first cluster in a white population. *Int. J. Cancer* **36**, 557–559.

125. Goldman-Leikin, R., Herst, C., Kies, M. *et al.* (1987). Human T-cell lymphotropic virus type 1-associated adult T-cell leukaemia/lymphoma in an atypical host. *Arch. Pathol. Lab. Med.* **111**, 1054–1056.

126. Levine, P., Blattner, W., Clark, J. *et al.* (1988). Geographic distribution of

HTLV-1 and identification of a new high risk population. *Int. J. Cancer* **42**, 7–12.

127. Robert-Guroff, M., Weiss, S., Giron, J. *et al.* (1986). Prevalence of antibodies to HTLV 1, 2 and 3 in IV drug users from an AIDS endemic region. *J. Am. Med. Assoc.* **255**, 3133–3137.

128. Tajima, K., Tominaga, S., Suchi, T. *et al.* (1982). Epidemiological analysis of the distribution of antibody to adult T-cell-leukaemia-virus-associated antigen: possible horizontal transmission of adult T-cell leukaemia virus. *Jpn. J. Cancer Res.* **73**, 893–901.

129. Rezza, G., Titti, F., Rossi, G. *et al.* (1988). Sex as a risk factor for HTLV-1 spread among IV drug abusers. *Lancet* **i**, 713.

130. Weber, J. Unpublished observations.

131. Komuro, A., Hayami, M., Fujii, H. *et al.* (1983). Vertical transmission of adult T-cell leukaemia virus. *Lancet* **i**, 240.

132. Nakano, S., Ando, Y., Ichjio, M. *et al.* (1984). Search for possible routes of vertical and horizontal transmission of adult T-cell leukaemia virus. *Jpn. J. Cancer Res.* **75**, 1044–1045.

133. Kotani, S., Yoshimoto, S., Yamoto, K. *et al.* (1986). Serial transmission of human T-cell leukaemia virus type I by blood transfusion in rabbits and its prevention by use of X-irradiated stored blood. *Int. J. Cancer* **37**, 843–847.

134. Hirose, S., Kotani, S., Uemura, Y. *et al.* (1988). Milk borne transmission of HTLV-1 in rabbits. *Virology* **162**, 487–489.

135. Yamanouchi, K., Kinoshita, K., Moriuchi, R. *et al.* (1985). Oral transmission of human T-cell leukaemia virus type I into a common marmoset (*Callithrix jacchus*) as an experimental model for milk-borne transmission. *Jpn J. Cancer Res.* **76**, 481–487.

136. Kinoshita, K., Hino, S., Amagaski, T. *et al.* (1984). Demonstration of adult T-cell leukaemia virus antigen in milk from three sero-positive mothers. *Jpn J. Cancer Res.* **75**, 103–105.

137. Hino, S., Sugiyama, H., Doi, H. *et al.* (1987). Breaking the cycle of HTLV-1 transmission via carrier mother's milk. *Lancet* **ii**, 158–159.

138. Ando, Y., Saito, K., Nakano, S. *et al.* (1989). Bottle feeding can prevent transmission of HTLV-1 from mothers to their babies. *J. Infect.* **19**, 25–29.

139. Hino, S., Kawamichi, T., Funakoshi, M. *et al.* (1984). Transfusion mediated spread of the human T-cell leukaemia virus in chronic haemodialysis patients in a heavily endemic area, Nagasaki. *Jpn. J. Cancer Res.* **75**, 1070–1075.

140. Okochi, K., Sato, H. and Hinuma, Y. (1984). A retrospective study on transmission of ATL virus by blood transfusion: seroconversion in recipients. *Vox Sang.* **46**, 245–253.

141. Agius, G., Biggar, R., Alexander, S. *et al.* (1988). Human T lymphotropic virus type I antibody patterns: evidence of difference by age and risk group. *J. Infect. Dis.* **158**, 1235–1244.

142. Greaves, M., Verbi, W., Tilley, R. *et al.* (1984). Human T-cell leukaemia virus (HTLV) in the United Kingdom. *Int. J. Cancer* **33**, 795–806.

143. Ueda, K., Kusuhara, K. and Tokugawa, K. (1988). Transmission of HTLV-1. *Lancet* **i**, 1163–1164.

144. Broder, S. (moderator) (1984). T-cell lymphoproliferative syndrome associated with HTLV. *Ann. Int. Med.* **100**, 543–557.

145. Bunn, P., Schechter, G., Jaffe, E. *et al.* (1983). Clinical course of retrovirus associated adult T-cell lymphoma in the US. *New Engl. J. Med.* **309**, 257–264.

146. Yamaguchi, K., Nishimura, H., Kohrogi, H. *et al.* (1983). A proposal for smouldering adult T-cell leukaemia: a clinicopathologic study of five cases. *Blood* **62**, 758–766.
147. Gessain, A., Barin, F., Vernant, J. *et al.* (1985). Antibodies to HTLV-1 in patients with tropical spastic paraparesis. *Lancet* **ii**, 407–409.
148. Montogomery, R., Cruickshank, E., Robertson, W. and McMenemy, W. (1964). Clinical and pathological observations in Jamaican neuropathy. A report of 206 cases. *Brain* **87**, 425–462.
149. Newton, M., Cruikshank, K., Miller, D. *et al.* (1987). Antibody to human T-lymphotropic virus type 1 in West Indian born UK residents with spastic paraparesis. *Lancet* **i**, 415–416.
150. Rodgers-Johnson, P., Gajdusek, D., Morgan, O. *et al.* (1985). HTLV-I and HTLV-III antibodies and tropical spastic paraparesis. *Lancet* **ii**, 1247–1248.
151. Osame, M., Usuku, K., Izumo, S. *et al.* (1986). HTLV-1 associated myelopathy, a new clinical entity. *Lancet* **i**, 1031–1032.
152. Osame, M., Igata, A., Usuku, K. *et al.* (1987). Mother to child transmission in HTLV-I associated myelopathy. *Lancet* **i**, 106.
153. Cartier-Rovirosa, L., Mora, C., Araya, F. *et al.* (1989). HTLV-1 positive TSP in a temperate zone. *Lancet* **i**, 556–557.
154. Annunziata, P., Fanetti, G., Giarratana, M. *et al.* (1987). HTLV-1 associated spastic paraparesis in an Italian woman. *Lancet* **ii**, 1393–1394.
155. Yoshida, M., Osame, M., Usuku, K. *et al.* (1987). Viruses detected in HTLV-1-associated myelopathy and ATL are identical on DNA blotting. *Lancet* **i**, 1085–1086.
156. Ceroni, M., Piccardo, D., Rodgers-Johnson, P. *et al.* (1988). Intra-thecal synthesis of IgG antibodies to HTLV-1 supports an aetiological role for HTLV-1 in TSP. *Ann. Neurol.* **23** Suppl: S 188–191.
157. Dalgleish, A., Richardson, J., Matutes, E. *et al.* (1988). HTLV-1 infection in tropical spastic paraparesis: lymphocyte culture and serologic response. *AIDS Res. Hum. Retrovir.* **4**, 475–485.
158. Morgan, O., Rodgers-Johnson, P., Gibbs, W. *et al.* (1987). Abnormal peripheral lymphocytes in tropical spastic paraparesis. *Lancet* **ii**, 403–404.
159. Bartholomew, C., Cleghorn, F., Charles, W. *et al.* (1986). HTLV-1 and tropical spastic paraparesis. *Lancet* **ii**, 99–100.
160. Tournier-Lasserve, E., Gout, O., Gessain, A. *et al.* (1987). HTLV-1, brain abnormalities on magnetic resonance imaging and relation with multiple sclerosis. *Lancet* **ii**, 49–50.
161. Mattson, D., McFarlin, D., Mora, C. and Zaninovic, V. (1987). Central-nervous-system lesions detected by magnetic resonance imaging in an HTLV-1 antibody positive symptomless individual. *Lancet* **ii**, 49.
162. Koprowski, H., DeFreitas, E., Harper, M. *et al.* (1985). Multiple sclerosis and human T-cell lymphotropic retroviruses. *Nature, Lond.* **318**, 154–160.
163. Reddy, P., Sandberg-Wollheim, M. and Mettus, R. (1989). Amplification and molecular cloning of HTLV-1 sequences from DNA of multiple sclerosis patients. *Science* **243**, 529–533.
164. Karpas, A., Kampf, U., Siden, A. *et al.* (1986). Lack of evidence for involvement of known human retroviruses in multiple sclerosis. *Nature, Lond.* **322**, 177–178.
165. Hauser, S., Aubert, C., Burks, J. *et al.* (1986). Analysis of human T-lymphotropic virus sequences in multiple sclerosis tissue. *Nature, Lond.* **322**, 176–177.

166. Bangham, C., Nightingale, S., Cruickshank, J. and Daenke, S. (1989). PCR analysis of DNA from MS patients for the presence of HTLV-1. *Science* **246**, 821.

167. Richardson, J., Wucherpfennig, K., Endo, N. *et al.* (1989). PCR analysis of DNA from MS patients for the presence of HTLV-1. *Science* **246**, 821–823.

168. Bartholomew, C., Blattner, W. and Cleghorn, F. (1987). Progression to AIDS in homosexual men co-infected with HIV-1 and HTLV-1 in Trinidad. *Lancet* **ii**, 1469.

169. Harper, M., Kaplan, M., Marselle, L. *et al.* (1986). Concomitant infection with HTLV-1 and HTLV-III in T8 lymphoproliferative disease. *New Engl. J. Med.* **315**, 1073–1078.

170. Mulin, G., Sheppell, A. and Mayer, L. (1988). Infection with HTLV-1 and HTLV-III in T8 lymphoproliferative disease. *New Engl. J. Med.* **316**, 1343.

171. Wiley, C., Neremberg, M., Cros, D. *et al.* (1989). HTLV-I polymyositis in a patient also infected by HIV. *New Engl. J. Med.* **320**, 992–995.

172. Morgan, O., Rodgers-Johnson, P., Mora, C. and Char, G. (1989). HTLV-1 and polymyositis in Jamaica. *Lancet* **ii**, 1184–1186.

173. Immamura, N., Inada, T. and Kuramoto, A. (1989). Multiple primary malignant neoplasms in patients with ATL. *Lancet* **i**, 219.

174. Tachibana, N., Okayama, A., Ishizaki, J. *et al.* (1988). Suppression of tuberculin skin reactivity in healthy HTLV-1 carriers from Japan. *Int. J. Cancer* **42**, 829–831.

175. Vernant, J., Buisson, G., Magdeleine, H. *et al.* (1988). T lymphocyte alveolitis, TSP and Sjögren's syndrome. *Lancet* **i**, 177.

176. Sugimoto, M., Nakashima, H., Watanabe, S. *et al.* (1987). T-lymphocyte alveolitis in HTLV-1 associated myelopathy. *Lancet* **ii**, 1220.

177. Pandolfi, F., Schriver, K., Scarselli, E. *et al.* (1987). HTLV-1 antibodies and lymphoproliferative disease of granular lymphocytes. *Lancet* **ii**, 1527.

178. Nishioka, K., Maruyama, I., Sato, K. *et al.* (1989). Chronic inflammatory arthropathy associated with HTLV-1. *Lancet* **ii**, 441.

179. Murphey, E., Hanchard, B., Figueroa, J. *et al.* (1989). Modelling the risk of ATL in patients infected by HTLV-1. *Int. J. Cancer* **43**, 250–253.

8 | The Molecular and Biological Properties of Human Herpesvirus 6 (HHV-6)

BRIAN J. THOMSON, MICHELLE E.D. MARTIN
and ROBERT W. HONESS

*Division of Virology, National Institute for Medical Research,
The Ridgeway, Mill Hill, London NW7 1AA, UK*

8.1 INTRODUCTION

Human herpesvirus 6 (HHV-6) was first isolated from the peripheral blood lymphocytes of six individuals with lymphoproliferative disorders, two of whom were also infected with human immunodeficiency virus (HIV) [1]. The virus, initially named human B-lymphotropic virus (HBLV), possessed the morphogenetic and structural features typical of the herpesvirus family but was antigenically distinct from other characterized primate herpesviruses. In addition, hybridization experiments showed no evidence of identity between selected regions of the HBLV/HHV-6 genome and other human herpesviruses [2]. Independent isolates of closely similar viruses have now been reported from different regions of Africa [3–6], Japan [7], Australia [8], South Africa [9] and the UK [10]. All isolates of this previously unrecognized human herpesvirus are now designated HHV-6. Evidence of infection with HHV-6 is very common in healthy adult populations of widely different geographical origin [11–13]. The virus has been unambiguously identified as the cause of exanthem subitum, a pyrexial illness of early infancy [7], and has been less convincingly linked with a number of other conditions of greater medical importance. In addition, prior infection with HHV-6 has been postulated as a cofactor in the progression of asymptomatic HIV-infected individuals to AIDS [14]. In this review we summarize current knowledge of the molecular and biological properties of HHV-6 and explore the potential role of the virus in human disease. We also briefly summarize some features of the herpesvirus family which form a necessary background to the study of HHV-6.

8.2 THE HERPESVIRUS FAMILY

All herpesviruses possess a single, double-stranded DNA genome packaged into a complex icosahedral nucleocapsid within the nuclei of

AIDS AND THE NEW VIRUSES
ISBN 0–12–200740–9

productively infected cells. Each nucleocapsid is then enclosed in a protein tegument and glycoprotein envelope to yield the infectious extracellular particle. In addition to these common structural elements, herpesviruses share essential features of replication and maturation. Virus-encoded proteins are necessary for replication of viral DNA and progeny genomes are cleaved from concatameric intermediates. These common features are, however, possessed by viruses with a remarkable diversity in a range of other biological and molecular properties.

The herpesvirus family may be divided into three sub-families — α-, β- and γ-herpesviruses — on the basis of differences in their host range and tissue distribution in acute and persistent infections *in vivo* and differences in host cell range and growth characteristics *in vitro*. The properties of each subfamily and the diseases with which they are associated are summarized in Table 8.1. Human herpesviruses are the most completely characterized members of each group. Productive infection with each of these viruses is cytocidal. Viral gene expression occurs in at least three sequential phases: immediate early (IE), delayed early (DE) and late. In addition, all herpesviruses share the ability to establish latent or persistent infection in which viral gene expression is highly restricted. Maintenance of the latent state is in part a function of the host immune system. Herpesviruses are important pathogens of immunocompromised hosts.

Herpesvirus genomes vary in size from 120 to 240 kilobases (kb) and in mean base composition from 32–75% (G+C). In addition, herpesviruses vary in the size and orientation within the genome of reiterated relatively G+C-rich DNA sequences. The complete nucleotide sequences of genomes from prototype strains of Epstein–Barr virus (EBV) [15], varicella zoster virus (VZV) [16], herpes simplex virus (HSV) [17] and human cytomegalovirus (HCMV) [18] are now available. Three principal conclusions can be drawn from the analysis of these sequences:

(1) All herpesviruses contain a subset of essential replicative and structural genes that are clearly homologous. These genes are arranged in blocks, the relative positions of which are a property of the virus subfamily.

(2) The similarities in the arrangements of homologous genes and in their protein sequences are significantly greater in comparisons between viruses of the same subfamily.

(3) Members of a subfamily possess groups of genes which occur within that subfamily and no other, and within some such groups some genes appear to be restricted to a particular virus species or group of closely related species.

Table 8.1   Classification of herpesviruses.

Subfamily	α-Herpesviruses	β-Herpesviruses	γ-Herpesviruses
Representative members	Herpes simplex virus (HSV-1 and HSV-2); varicella zoster virus (VZV)	Human cytomegalovirus (HCMV)	Epstein–Barr virus (EBV)
Host range *In vivo*	Variable	Narrow, restricted to host species	Narrow, normally restricted to host species
In vitro	Wide	Fibroblasts	Lymphoblastoid cells occasionally epithelial cells and fibroblasts
Latency	Terminally differentiated ganglia	? Lymphoreticular cells	Lymphoid tissue ? immature epithelial cells
Reproductive cycle *In vitro*	Short (8–14 h)	Long (48–96 h)	Long (36–60 h)
Disease associations	Primary infection of epithelial cells (HSV); chicken pox (VZV); shingles (VZV)	Normally asymptomatic primary infection. Neurological disease in neonates	Normally asymptomatic primary infection. "Glandular fever syndrome" in late primary infection
	Disseminated infection of immuno-compromised hosts	Disseminated infection of immuno-compromised hosts	Lymphomas and nasopharyngeal carcinoma

It is therefore clear that the conserved core of replicative and structural genes has been derived from a common progenitor and areas of divergence from collinearity between viruses of different subfamilies are frequently demarcated by the presence of reiterated DNA-sequences. The nature of the adaptive and non-adaptive forces which have operated in the divergent evolution of these viruses from the ancestral genome and the interaction between the current sets of molecular and biological properties of herpesviruses are fundamental issues. The study of HHV-6 will both establish the intrinsic importance of this virus to human disease and further explore the relationships between the molecular phylogeny and biological properties of herpesviruses.

8.3   GROWTH CHARACTERISTICS AND CELLULAR TROPISM OF HHV-6

The original description of HHV-6 suggested that the virus infected only freshly isolated B cells and led to the suggestion of HBLV as a suitable label. It is now clear that this original isolate and all subsequently characterized strains of HHV-6 replicate preferentially in the PHA-stimulated T lymphocytes of human umbilical cord or adult peripheral blood (Figs 8.1, 8.2). In addition, a number of isolates can be routinely propagated in human T cell lines [4, 13, 19]. The infectious progeny of most isolates remain cell associated, but significant concentrations of cell-free infectious virus are generated by certain strains of HHV-6 which have been passaged extensively *in vitro* [13, 19]. Cell lines of B cell, megakaryocyte and glial cell origin can also support the replication of some isolates of HHV-6 [4, 19]. The molecular basis for these differences in cellular tropism and growth characteristics has not yet been determined. It is clear, however, that there is an absolute requirement for T cell activation to achieve productive infection, and that the majority of cells infected *in vitro* [20, 21] and *in vivo* [22] express the CD4 surface antigen. Lusso and colleagues have also proposed that the majority of cells supporting viral replication *in vitro* bear markers characteristic of immature T cells, i.e. they do not express the CD3/T cell receptor complex or the IL-2 receptor but express CD2 and coexpress CD4 and CD8. In contrast, Takahashi found HHV-6 replicating *in vitro* in fully mature cells which were predominantly CD3+ and CD4+ and CD8−. The precise role that the CD4 surface antigen plays in mediating infection with HHV-6 has not yet been established. A panel of anti-CD4 monoclonal antibodies did not block HHV-6 infection of CD4+ T cell lines [23].

There is, as yet, no evidence to identify the site of latent or persistent infection with HHV-6.

8.4   MORPHOLOGY AND MORPHOGENESIS

Electron microscopy of thin sections of cells productively infected with HHV-6 readily demonstrates high concentrations of the mature and immature forms of the virus particle characteristic of herpesvirus morphogenesis. Nuclei of infected cells contain both "empty" and "full" nucleocapsids with a diameter of 95–100 nm which can be negatively stained to reveal the typical 162 capsomer icosahedral structure [24]. Capsids can be seen budding through the inner nuclear membrane to yield enveloped particles without a prominent tegument. Mature enveloped virus with a prominent tegument and a diameter of 160–210 nm accumulates in cytoplasmic vacuoles and at the extracellular surface of infected cells. In addition, high concentrations of full capsids surrounded by an electron-dense layer of presumed tegument are observed free in the cytoplasm and apparently in the process of envelopment by budding into cytoplasmic vesicles. This feature of the

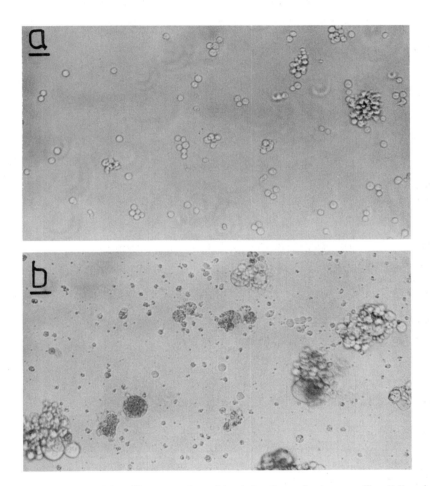

Fig. 8.1 Cytopathic effects produced by infection of a human T cell line (J-JHAN, a clonal derivative of JURKAT) with the U1102 isolate of HHV-6. Low-power fields (× 100) of unstained specimens of uninfected cells (a) and cells from a culture 7 days after infection with HHV-6 (b).

(a): total inf. cell DNA

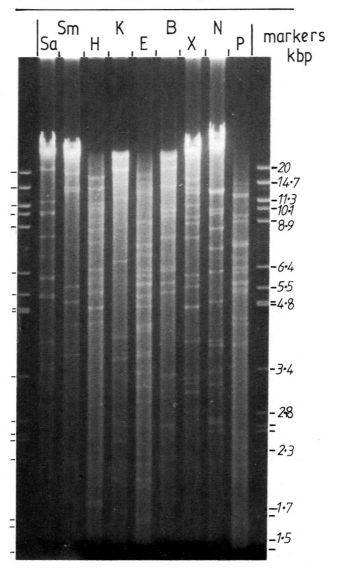

Fig. 8.2 Direct detection of restriction fragments of HHV-6 (U1102) DNA in digests of DNA from total infected cord-blood lymphocytes (panel a) and from crude "nuclear" (n) and cytoplasmic (c) fractions from infected cord-blood lymphocytes. Purified high molecular weight DNA samples were digested with a range of restriction enzymes (SallI, Sa; Smal, Sm; HindlII, H; KpnI, K; EcoRI, E; BamHI, B; Xhol, X; Nrul, N; and PstI, P) and the resulting

DNA from "cytoplasmic" (c) and
(b): "nuclear"(n) fractions

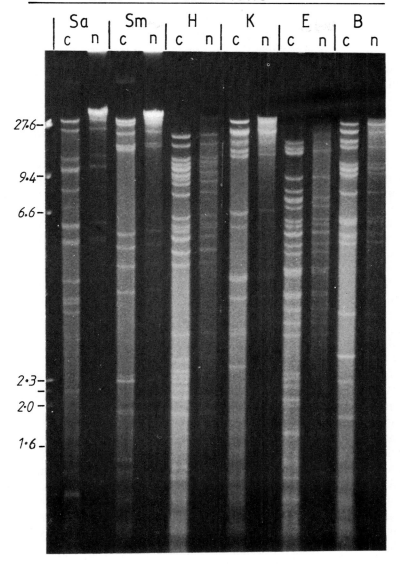

fragments separated by electrophoresis through 0.6% agarose gels in a tris-borate-EDTA buffer (3 V/cm for (a) 40 or (b) 30 h). Gels were stained with ethidium bromide, irradiated with ultraviolet light and the fluorescent images photographed. Fragments arising from HHV-6 DNA are readily visible in all digests.

maturation of HHV-6 is similar to observations made with a number of other herpesviruses — notably herpesvirus of frogs [25], turkeys [26], herpesvirus saimiri [27], and cytomegalovirus [28] — and has been interpreted to suggest a distinct pathway of cytoplasmic envelopment. There is, however, no evidence to identify these structures as products of assembly rather than dis-assembly and their presence may represent the failure of the super-infection exclusion mechanism and abortive re-entry rather than an unusual pathway of maturation and egress.

8.5   THE DETECTION OF HHV-6 IN NORMAL POPULATIONS

Studies using indirect and anticomplementary immunofluorescence tests have indicated that up to 70% of an unselected adult population are seropositive for HHV-6 and that the majority acquire the infection within the first year of life [11, 13]. These tests use infected cell lines and peripheral or cord blood mononuclear cells as substrate. A positive reaction with a minimum dilution of human serum of 1:50 appears to be a specific measure of antibody to HHV-6. There is no correlation with titres of antibody to other human herpesviruses [11, 29] and all individuals from whom HHV-6 can be isolated score positively. In addition, cross-adsorption of HHV-6-positive sera with preparations of cells infected with other human herpesviruses does not remove reactivity to HHV-6. The prevalence and titre of antibody to HHV-6 is highest in children and young adults, and females over the age of 15 have higher mean antibody titres than age-matched male controls ([11]; C. Lopez *et al.*, personal communication). A more sensitive competitive radioimmunoassay for HHV-6 antibody suggests a seroprevalence of up to 90% in a healthy adult population (J. Fox, personal communication).

A simultaneous rise in antibody titres to HHV-6 and HCMV has been recorded in small numbers of individuals, from some of whom HCMV has been isolated [30, 31]. These results may represent co-reactivation of these two viruses. A recent study has, however, demonstrated that rising antibody titres to HHV-6 in a small proportion of individuals who had recently undergone organ transplantation is cross-adsorbed by HCMV antigens (G. Christofinis, personal communication). HHV-6 and HCMV antigens expressed during reactivation may therefore cross-react in certain hosts. Recombinant HHV-6 proteins have now been expressed ([32]; E. Littler, personal communication) and monoclonal antibodies have been raised to HHV-6 antigens [33, 34]. The use of such materials should provide the basis of specific methods for the detection of HHV-6.

We have recently developed the polymerase chain reaction (PCR) as a highly sensitive and specific means of detecting the presence of the genome of HHV-6 and other herpesviruses in blood and tissues. Preliminary results indicate that HHV-6 DNA can be detected in the blood and saliva of healthy adults. Sequences amplified from the EBV genome can be readily demonstrated in both blood and saliva of the majority of seropositive adults (Fig. 8.3).

8.6 DISEASE ASSOCIATIONS OF HHV-6

There is now unequivocal evidence that primary infection with HHV-6 is associated with exanthem subitum (roseola infantum), a self-limiting pyrexial illness of early infancy [7, 35]. The development of this disease can be clearly correlated with both seroconversion to HHV-6 and the isolation of virus from cultures of peripheral blood mononuclear cells. A remarkably high proportion of circulating mononuclear cells carry the virus during the febrile phase of the illness (10 000–200 000 infected cells/10^6 mononuclear cells).

The rapid increase in the prevalence of antibody to HHV-6 during the first year of life strongly suggests that the principal route of transmission is from mother to child. In a study of infants born to HTLV-1-infected mothers the time and frequency of seroconversion to HHV-6 and the incidence of exanthem subitum in those infants who were breast fed did not differ from those who were bottle fed (K. Yaminishi, personal communication, and 13th International Herpesvirus Workshop). A single Australian study has consistently isolated HHV-6 from the saliva of healthy adults [8]. A number of other laboratories in different geographical areas, however, have not yet reproduced these findings (C. Lopez, personal communication). It is possible that HHV-6 is reactivated and secreted during pregnancy and/or the post-natal period. Studies of saliva samples and the antibody profile of pregnant and lactating women will clarify this issue. A preliminary study has demonstrated IgM antibody to HHV-6 in 10 of 32 pregnant women and in 2 of 120 controls (J. Fox and R. Tedder, personal communication). Late primary infection with HHV-6 has been associated with mild febrile illness characterized by cervical lymphadenopathy, occasionally accompanied by rash resembling exanthem subitum [36, 37].

A role for HHV-6 has been postulated in the post-viral fatigue syndrome ([38]; R. Read, personal communication). This syndrome, also known as myalgic encephalomyelitis (ME), is a heterogenous group of conditions which may have in common an acute onset and a protracted

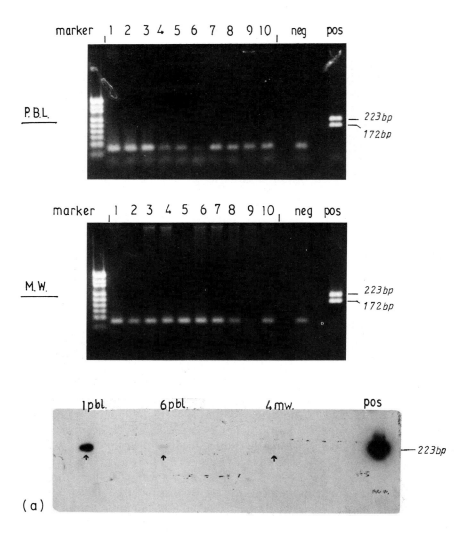

Fig. 8.3 Detection of the genomes of HHV-6 (a) and EBV (b) in blood and mouth-washings from normal adults by the use of primer-directed *in vitro* amplification with the polymerase chain reaction (PCR). DNA was extracted using conventional methods from the peripheral blood mononuclear cells and mouth-washings of 30 healthy adults. Oligonucleotides (25-mers) were chosen to prime synthesis of a 223 bp product from the spliced ORF of the HHV-6 genome and a 175 bp product from the analogous region of the EBV genome. PCR was performed for 40 cycles (1 min at 94°C; 1 min at 65°C; 2 min at 72°C) using approximately 500 ng of DNA as substrate in each reaction. One fifth of the final reaction volume was electrophoresed in 2% agarose gels, stained with ethidium bromide and the products visualized by UV transillumination. The PCR products were then transferred in 0.4 M NaOH onto nylon membranes and hybridized with an oligonucleotide probe

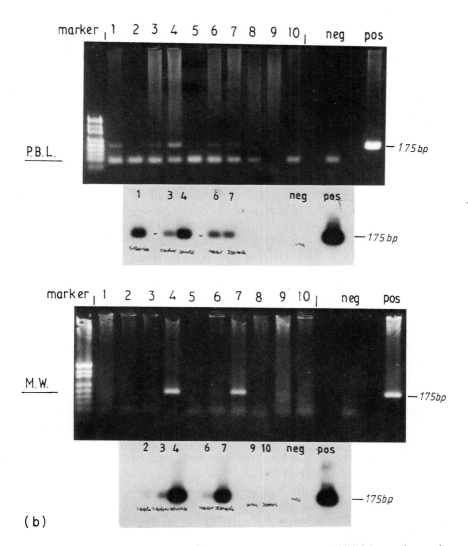

marker 1 2 3 4 5 6 7 8 9 10 neg pos

P.B.L.

—175bp

1 3 4 6 7 neg pos

—175bp

marker 1 2 3 4 5 6 7 8 9 10 neg pos

M.W.

—175bp

2 3 4 6 7 9 10 neg pos

—175bp

(b)

to sequences internal to the primers of the EBV and HHV-6 products. In these experiments none of the blood or saliva samples tested produced an HHV-6-specific product visible on an ethidium bromide gel. Two of the peripheral blood samples and three mouth-wash samples became positive on probing with the "internal" oligonucleotide. Each of the individuals from whom the positive samples were obtained was seropositive for HHV-6. A majority of EBV seropositive individuals were PCR positive as assessed both by visualization of EBV-specific bands on ethidium bromide and oligonucleotide probing. (The results of amplification of HHV-6 and EBV sequences from the blood and saliva of 10 individuals are illustrated.)

course characterized by myalgia, fatigue and mood disturbance [39]. Sporadic and epidemic forms have been described and persistent or recrudescent viral infections are a plausible cause. Komaroff and colleagues described 51 individuals with fatigue syndrome in whom antibody titres to HHV-6 were higher than in age-matched controls. In addition, Read and colleagues found that 37 patients who fitted an independent definition of the syndrome had a higher prevalence and titre of HHV-6 antibody than age- and sex-matched controls. In contrast, Wakefield *et al.* [40] found no difference in the antibody profile to HHV-6 in groups of patients and controls and C. Lopez *et al.* (personal communication) found that although titres of antibody to HHV-6 were elevated in comparison to controls, the magnitude of this elevation was no greater than that of antibody to many other viruses. The potential role of HHV-6 in this group of conditions cannot be established until there is a clear and consistently applied definition of the syndrome with which evidence of infection with HHV-6 can be correlated.

A number of attempts have been made to link HHV-6 with lymphoproliferative diseases. HHV-6 has been demonstrated by either *in situ* hybridization or Southern blotting and hybridization in the DNA from a minority of large cell follicular B cell lymphomas and Burkitt's lymphomas [41]; two B cell lymphomas associated with Sjögrens syndrome [42, 43]; lymphocytes undergoing "atypical" polyclonal proliferation [44] and in the lymph node of a single patient with sarcoidosis [45]. The presence of HHV-6 DNA is, however, not invariably associated with any of these diseases. HHV-6 antigens have also been shown to be expressed in the cervical lymph nodes of a number of individuals with lymphoproliferative diseases not necessarily involving cervical nodes [46]. Interpreting the significance of such associations is rendered difficult by the high prevalence of HHV-6 and the likely propensity of the virus to reactivate in immunocompromised hosts. Thirty continuous cell lines from human T and B cell neoplasias (including samples of EBV+ and EBV− Burkitt tumour cell lines) and DNA from lymph nodes and peripheral blood mononuclear cells from patients with active B and T cell non-Hodgkin's lymphomas did not contain HHV-6 DNA sequences detectable by Southern blotting and hybridization (U. Gompels, personal communication). No consistent link has therefore been demonstrated between HHV-6 and any lymphoproliferative disease. The definition of the latent site of HHV-6 and the nature of viral gene expression within that site will permit a more informed assessment of the potential role of HHV-6 in chronic and neoplastic disease in adults.

The potential of HHV-6 to interact with HIV is an area of significant current interest. It is striking that the majority of HHV-6 isolates from adults have been obtained from the peripheral blood mononuclear cells of HIV-infected individuals. Both viruses selectively infect CD4+ lymphocytes and require host cell activation for full viral gene expression. HHV-6 and HIV can co-infect the same cell *in vitro* [21]. HHV-6, in common with other herpesviruses [47, 48], is capable of transactivating the HIV LTR linked to the chloramphenicol acetyl transferase gene [49], and has additionally been shown to accelerate HIV gene expression and CD4 cell death in culture co-infected with both viruses [21]. This transactivating function is mediated by binding of factors induced or specified by HHV-6 to the enhancer region of the HIV LTR [14]. There is therefore convincing evidence for a molecular and cellular interaction between HHV-6 and HIV *in vitro*. PCR studies indicate that the proportion of circulating T cells which harbour the HIV provirus in asymptomatic HIV-infected individuals is much higher than previously believed, and may approach 1 in 100 cells [50] — although virus detected by PCR may be defective [51]. It is likely that high numbers of circulating mononuclear cells carry HHV-6 during productive infection. An interaction between HHV-6 in the lytic cycle and HIV is therefore plausible and merits further investigation. The potential of these two viruses to interact in their latent state cannot be explored until the site of latent infection with HHV-6 and the nature of viral gene expression within that site have been established. Preliminary epidemiological studies do not support a role for previous infection with HHV-6 in the progression of asymptomatic HIV-infected individuals to AIDS [12, 52]. The recent demonstration, however, that prior infection with HCMV accelerates the development of AIDS in HIV-infected haemophiliacs, suggests that the role of HHV-6 in this context remains an important issue [53].

8.7   THE HHV-6 GENOME

The HHV-6 genome is a linear double-stranded molecule of approximately 170 kb in length estimated by migration of unit length genomes in field inversion gels (Fig. 8.4) and summation of endonuclease restriction fragments (R.W. Honess and P.W. Pellet, personal communication). The mean mononucleotide composition is estimated to be 42–43% (G+C) by buoyant density in caesium chloride. Mapping of endonuclease restriction sites and cross-hybridization experiments performed on two different isolates of HHV-6 (Zaire isolate Z29 studied by P.W. Pellet and colleagues and Ugandan isolate U1102 studied in this laboratory) indicate that the genomes are homologous and collinear for most of their length. There are, however, regions of marked polymorphism of endonuclease recognition sites. Endonuclease restriction mapping and hybridization experiments have led to the development by Pellet and colleagues of a model for the gross structure of HHV-6 Z29 (Fig. 8.5). Independent data generated by mapping the U1102 genome are consistent with this model. The genome of the Z29 strain is composed of large-scale direct repeat units at each terminus of approximately 13.2 kb in length, with an intervening unique sequence of approximately 141 kb. Clones which represent portions of one end of the terminal duplications of HHV-6 U1102 have been sequenced and shown to be relatively G+C rich (M.A. Craxton and B.J. Thomson, unpublished observations). Interpretation of the pattern produced by hybridization of terminal clones to HHV-6 U1102 DNA demands that the repeat units are linked to unique sequence in more than the two predicted ways. Pellet has obtained evidence of a specific deletion of one of the junctions of unique and repeat sequence occurring in a discrete subpopulation of his prototype virus which provides an explanation for these observations. The data generated by mapping these two different isolates is therefore entirely consistent with the suggested model. This structure of the HHV-6 genome would be unique among human herpesviruses and most closely resembles the structures proposed for genomes from channel catfish virus and a subset of equine cytomegaloviruses [54].

The original studies of the HHV-6 genome did not demonstrate cross-hybridization with selected fragments of other human herpesviruses [2]. HHV-6 has since been shown to share a short reiterated sequence (GGGTTA) with the avian herpesvirus responsible for Marek's disease [55]. These results are unlikely to represent any uniquely close relationship between the two viruses. However, selected regions of the HHV-6 genome have been shown to hybridize under stringent conditions to HCMV [56]. Endonuclease restriction fragments of U1102 have been used as substrate for small- and large-scale nucleic acid sequencing of the viral genome. The results demonstrate that the cross-hybridization of HHV-6 with HCMV is a consequence of sequences encoding homologous genes and is indicative of a more extensive and important relationship between the two viruses. A contiguous sequence 21.8 kb in length from the unique region of the U1102 genome has been completed [57]. Analysis of the DNA sequence and amino acid sequence of predicted gene products has provided the most comprehensive basis for comparison with other herpesviruses. The sequence has a mean base composition of 41% (G+C) and the frequency of each dinucleotide pair is consistent with this mononucleotide composition. This HHV-6 sequence therefore shows no evidence of the CpG dinucleotide suppression observed throughout the genomes of the lymphotropic herpesviruses EBV and

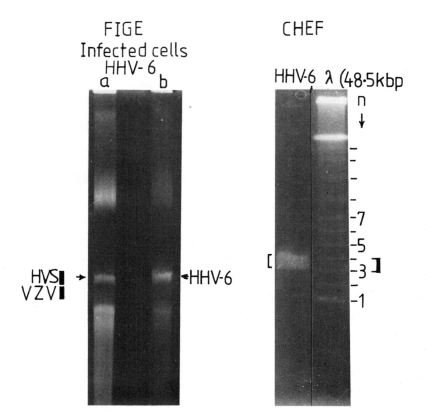

Fig. 8.4 Estimates of the size of the HHV-6 (strain U1102) genome by field-inversion gel electrophoresis (FIGE) and contour-clamped homogeneous-field electrophoresis (CHEF). Samples of intact HHV-6-infected cord-blood lymphocytes (a and b) were sedimented, washed in PBS and set into low gelling-temperature agarose blocks (final concentration of 0.5% Sigma "low-melting point" agarose in PBS). The blocks were then incubated in a buffer containing 0.5 mg/ml of protease-K and 0.5% SDS for >24 h at 25°C, washed and equilibrated with 0.5 × tris-borate-EDTA buffer and then set into a 1.0% "low-melting point" agarose gel and separated by field-inversion gel electrophoresis (FIGE; 200 V/80 mA/9 s forward, 3 s reverse for 12 h at 12°C). The arrowed band is virus-specific, it migrates together with unit-length DNA from herpesvirus saimiri (HVS, ~ 160 kbp) and slower than unit-length DNA from varicella zoster virus (VZV, 124 kbp). Virus particles sedimented from the cytoplasmic fraction of HHV-6 infected cells were resuspended, set into agarose blocks and digested (as above) and the washed blocks set into a 1.0% agarose gel and separated by CHEF together with a sample of concatameric DNA from bacteriophage λ (i.e. 48.5 kbp × n). The HHV-6 DNA migrates just ahead of the $n=4$ band and behind the $n=3$ band of the λ-ladder (i.e. >145.5 and <194.0 kbp). Mean estimates of the size of the HHV-6 (U1102) genome based on FIGE and CHEF — separations of this type are ~ 160 kbp.

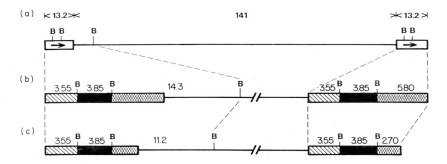

Fig. 8.5 Model for the structure of the HHV-6 Z29 genome (courtesy of P.W. Pellet and colleagues). The genome is proposed to consist of large-scale direct repeat units of approximately 13.2 kb in length situated at each terminus, with an intervening unique sequence of approximately 141 kb (a). A specific deletion at the left-hand junction of unique and repeat sequence occurs in a proportion of the virus population (b and c). Hybridization of the BamH1 clone spanning this junction (BamH1 sites marked B) to BamH1 digest of virion DNA will detect four discrete fragments (14.3 and 5.8 kb, 11.2 and 2.7 kb). Hybridization of this clone to digests of DNA extracted from infected cells, in which a proportion of the virus population will be present as concatameric intermediates, will produce a more complex pattern. This model is consistent with independent data generated by the study of a Ugandan isolate of HHV-6 (U1102) (R.W. Honess, M.E.D. Martin and B.J. Thomson).

HVS [58]. Seventeen complete open reading frames (ORFs) and part of another have been identified. The arrangement of these ORFs most closely resembles the arrangement of the homologous genes in the HCMV genome (Fig. 8.6). In particular, the major capsid genes of both HHV-6 and HCMV are inverted relative to the orientation observed in the genomes of HSV, VZV, EBV and HVS. Nine of the 17 ORFs find homologues in each of the other human herpesviruses and are identifiable as family-specific genes. These genes include homologues of the alkaline exonuclease and phosphotransferase genes, the spliced ORF of unknown function and the gene encoding the major capsid protein. The sequence of these genes in HHV-6 U1102 is most similar to that of the homologous genes of HCMV and the degree of this similarity is comparable to that found between homologous genes in viruses belonging to the same subfamily. In addition, HHV-6 contained three ORFs that had homologues in HCMV only. These genes are likely to be subfamily-specific and further identify HHV-6 as a member of the β-herpesvirus subfamily. Three of the HHV-6 ORFs had no identifiable homologues in the genomes of other human herpesviruses. No function has yet been

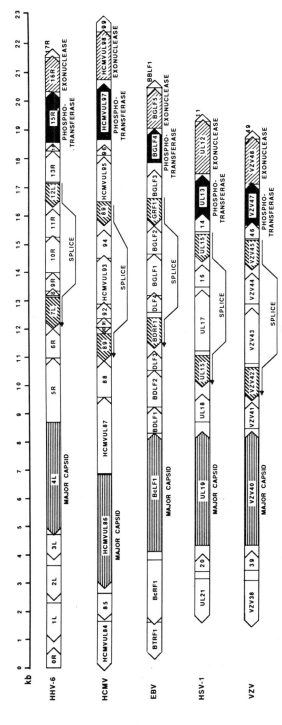

Fig. 8.6 Comparisons of the organization of coding sequences for some conserved and non-conserved genes in the genome of HHV-6 with the organization of homologous regions from the genomes of human cyto-megalovirus (HCMV), Epstein–Barr virus (EBV), herpes simplex virus type 1 (HSV-1) and varicella zoster virus (VZV). A sequence of 21.8 kbp from the HHV-6 (U1102) genome was determined and predicted to contain 12 open reading frames on the forward-strand (i.e. "rightward" frames, 0R to 17R) and 6 open reading frames on the complementary strand ("leftward" frames, 1L to 12L). Comparisons of the protein sequences encoded by these open reading frames with products predicted from the completed sequences of genomes from HCMV (strain AD169; [18]), EBV [15], HSV-1 [17] and VZV [16] showed that this region of the HHV-6 genome was homologous to the region of HCMV encoding UL84–UL99, and to the corresponding regions of the other human herpesviruses (e.g. UL21 to UL11 of HSV-1) and thus contained coding sequences (filled blocks, UL15 of HSV-1) to alkaline exonuclease (cross-hatched, UL12 of HSV-1). Pairwise comparisons of these protein sequences showed that the products of the HHV-6 genome were significantly more closely related to those of HCMV than to the products of the other human herpesviruses. In addition, HHV-6 and HCMV have in common an inversion of the major capsid protein gene and its 5' neighbour (4L and 5R in HHV-6; UL86 and UL87 in HCMV) with respect to the spliced gene, relative to the organization of the homologous genes of EBV, HSV-1 and VZV (data from Lawrence *et al.* [57]).

assigned to the proteins putatively encoded by these genes. The degree of relatedness of each of the human herpesviruses and herpesvirus saimiri, a γ-herpesvirus of primates, is illustrated by comparison of the predicted amino acid sequence of the spliced ORF (Table 8.2). Nucleic acid sequencing of another region of the U1102 genome has identified linked genes which have homologues in HCMV only (S. Efstathiou, personal communication, and 14th International Herpesvirus Workshop) and further suggests that HHV-6 does not contain the MHC class I related gene recently discovered in HCMV [59]. Sequence information has also been obtained from other HHV-6 isolates (P.W. Pellet, 14th International Herpes Virus Workshop, and S.Z. Salahuddin, personal communication). The results of large-scale sequencing of the HHV-6 genome clearly indicate that the virus is most similar to HCMV and is likely to belong to the β-herpesvirus subfamily. The HCMV genome may therefore be used as a model to predict the likely position within the HHV-6 genome of homologous genes. In addition, the similarity of biological properties of viruses belonging to the same subfamily suggests that HCMV may provide a paradigm for the exploration of the biological properties of HHV-6 and their likely relevance to clinical disease.

8.8   HHV-6 PROTEINS

The study of HHV-6 specific proteins has been hindered by the slow and asynchronous growth of most viral isolates *in vitro* and the apparent inability of HHV-6 to shut off host cell protein synthesis. A single published study has used a combination of ^{35}S methionine and ^{3}H

Table 8.2 Percentage amino acid similarity observed in comparisons between a portion of exon 2 of the conserved "spliced" gene from representative herpesviruses.

Group	Virus	HHV-6	HCMV	EBV	HVS	HSV-1	VZV
α	VZV	46	48	41	27	68	(100)
α	HSV-1	47	47	46	34	(100)	
γ	HVS	44	36	68	(100)		
γ	EBV	44	49	(100)			
β	HCMV	66	(100)				
	HHV-6	(100)					
%G+C[a]		43%	57%	60%	36%	68%	46%

[a] Mean %(G+C) of corresponding genome.

glucosamine labelling and Western blotting and immunoprecipitation to identify proteins encoded by the GS strain of HHV-6 in a human T cell line [33]. Polyclonal rabbit antibodies and human sera from individuals infected with HHV-6 identified more than 30 proteins and seven glycoproteins. Individuals with high titre antibody to other herpesviruses did not recognize the majority of these products but consistently precipitated a common 135 kD polypeptide. Monoclonal antibodies to HHV-6 infected cells identified three distinct sets of glycoproteins. None of these proteins has yet been further characterized.

The production of recombinant HHV-6 proteins has been so far limited by the lack of information on the major virus-specific immunogens and by available sequence information to permit the identification of ORFs suitable for expression. A 130 kD product of a subclone of GS has been expressed in baculovirus [32]. The relationship of this protein to sequences recognized in other herpesviruses is not yet clear. The major capsid protein has been expressed in whole or in part in *E. coli* (E. Littler, personal communication). The full length 135 kD polypeptide was immunogenic in mice but reacted only weakly in Western blot with sera from HHV-6-infected individuals, and it seems unlikely that this protein will provide the basis for a sensitive or specific immunoassay for antibody to HHV-6.

A DNA polymerase activity has been identified in cells infected with HHV-6 [60]. This polymerase has a similar sensitivity to inhibition by pyrophosphate analogues as other herpesvirus DNA polymerases, but shows a unique pattern of sensitivity to nucleoside triphosphate analogues. HHV-6 is inhibited *in vitro* much more effectively by gancyclovir than acyclovir [61, 62].

8.9   CONCLUSION

HHV-6 is a clearly distinct member of the herpesvirus family. It is the causative agent of exanthem subitum. No unambiguous link has yet been established between infection with HHV-6 and any other disease, although the molecular and biological properties of the virus suggest its potential role as a cofactor in the depletion of CD4 lymphocytes critical in the progression of AIDS in HIV-infected individuals. HHV-6 can clearly establish lytic infection in lymphocytes and has therefore been regarded as likely to belong to the subfamily of γ- or lymphotropic herpesviruses, such as EBV. However, these viruses are characterized by their ability to maintain latent or non-productive infection and highly restricted gene expression within a population of dividing lymphoid cells. No evidence yet available demonstrates that HHV-6 possesses this ability. The available evidence clearly indicates that HHV-6 is more closely related genetically to HCMV than to any other characterized human herpesvirus. The correlation between the molecular and biological properties of herpesviruses within the same subfamily suggests that HCMV should provide a useful model with which to explore the biological properties of HHV-6. In particular, reactivation of latent HHV-6 infection in immunocompromised individuals and recipients of allogeneic organ transplants may prove to be important. Additionally, determination of the molecular basis for divergence in properties between the apparently collinear genomes of HHV-6 and HCMV may shed valuable light on the phylogeny of herpesviruses.

REFERENCES

1. Salahuddin, S.Z., Ablashi, D.V., Markham, P.D. *et al.* (1986). *Science* **234**, 596–600.
2. Josephs, S.F., Salahuddin, S.Z., Ablashi, D.V., Schachter, F., Wong-Staal, F. and Gallo, R.C. (1986). *Science* **234**, 601–603.
3. Downing, R.G., Sewankambo, N., Serwadda, D. *et al.* (1987). *Lancet* **ii**, 390.
4. Tedder, R.S., Briggs, M., Cameron, C.H., Honess, R., Robertson, D. and Whittle, H. (1987). *Lancet* **ii**, 390–392.
5. Lopez, C., Pellet, P., Stewart, J. *et al.* (1988). *J. Infect. Dis.* **157**, 1271–1273.
6. Agut, H., Guetard, D., Collandre, H. *et al.* (1988). *Lancet* **i**, 712.
7. Yamanishi, K., Okuno, T., Shiraki, K. *et al.* (1988). *Lancet* **i**, 1065–1067.
8. Pietroboni, G.R., Harnett, G.B., Bucens, M.R. and Honess, R.W. (1988). *Lancet* **i**, 1059.
9. Becker, W.B., Engelbrecht, S., Becker, M.L.B. *et al.* (1989). *Lancet* **i**, 41.
10. Ward, K.N., Gray, J.J. and Efstathiou, S. (1989). *J. Med. Virol.* **28**, 69–72.
11. Briggs, M., Fox, J. and Tedder, R.S. (1988). *Lancet* **i**, 1058–1059.
12. Brown, N.A., Kovacs, A., Lui, C.-R., Hur, C., Zaia, J.A. and Mosley, J.W. (1988). *Lancet* **ii**, 1146.
13. Okuno, T., Takahashi, K., Balachandra, K. *et al.* (1989). *J. Clin. Microbiol.* **27**, 651–653.
14. Ensoli, B., Lusso, P., Schachter, F. *et al.* (1989). *EMBO J.* **8**, 3019–3027.
15. Baer, R., Bankier, A.T., Biggin, M.D. *et al.* (1984). *Nature, Lond.* **310**, 207–211.
16. Davison, A.J. and Scott, J.E. (1986). *J. Gen. Virol.* **67**, 1759–1816.
17. Perry, L.J. and McGeoch, D.J. (1988). *J. Gen. Virol.* **69**, 2831–2846.
18. Chee, M.S., Bankier, A.T., Beck, S. *et al.* (1990). *Curr. Topics Microbiol. Immunol.* (in press).
19. Ablashi, D.V., Salahuddin, S.Z., Josephs, S.F., Imam, F., Lusso, P. and Gallo, R.C. (1987). *Nature, Lond.* **329**, 207.
20. Lusso, P., Markham, P.D., Tschachler, R. *et al.* (1988). *J. Exp. Med.* **167**, 1659–1670.

21. Lusso, P., Ensoli, B., Markham, P.D. *et al.* (1989). *Nature, Lond.* **337**, 370–373.
22. Takahashi, K., Sonoda, S., Higashi, K. *et al.* (1989). *J. Virol.* **63**, 3161–3163.
23. Lusso, P., Gallo, R.C., De Rocco, S.E. and Markham, P.D. (1989). *Lancet* **i**, 730–731.
24. Biberfeld, P., Kramarsky, B., Salahuddin, S.Z. and Gallo, R.C. (1987). *J. Natl Cancer Inst.* **79**, 933–941.
25. Stackpole, C.W. and Mizell, M. (1968). *Virology* **36**, 63–72.
26. Hinshaw, V.L. and Mora, E.C. (1980). *Poultry Sci.* **59**, 258–266.
27. Tralka, T.S., Costa, J. and Robson, A. (1977). *Virology* **80**, 158–165.
28. Papadimitriou, J.M., Shellam, G.R. and Roberton, T.A. (1984). *J. Gen. Virol.* **65**, 1979–1990.
29. Morris, D.J., Littler, E., Jordan, D. and Arrand, J.R. (1988). *Lancet* **ii**, 1425–1426.
30. Larcher, C., Huemer, H.P., Margreiter, R. and Dierich, M.P. (1988). *Lancet* **ii**, 963–964.
31. Irving, W.L., Cunningham, A.L., Keogh, A. and Chapman, J.R. (1988). *Lancet* **ii**, 630–631.
32. Fung, M.-C., Chiu, K.Y.M., Weber, T., Chang, T.-W. and Chang, N.T. (1988). *J. Virol. Meth.* **19**, 33–42.
33. Balachandran, N., Amelse, R.E., Zhou, W.W. and Chang, C.K. (1989). *J. Virol.* **63**, 2835–2840.
34. Shiraki, K., Okuno, T., Yamanishi, K. and Takahashi, M. (1989). *Virus Res.* **13**, 173–178.
35. Takahashi, K., Sonoda, S., Kawakami, K. *et al.* (1988). *Lancet* **i**, 1463.
36. Niederman, J.C., Liu, C.-R., Kaplan, M.H. and Brown, N.A. (1988). *Lancet* **ii**, 817–818.
37. Kirchesch, H., Mertens, T., Burkhardt, U., Kruppenbacher, J.P., Hoffken, A. and Eggers, H.J. (1988). *Lancet* **ii**, 273–274.
38. Komaroff, A.L., Saxinger, C., Buchwald, D., Geiger, A. and Gallo, R.C. (1988). *Clin. Res.* **36**, 743 A.
39. Strauss, S.E. (1988). *J. Infect. Dis.* **157**, 405–411.
40. Wakefield, D., Lloyd, A., Dwyer, J., Salahuddin, S. and Ablashi, D.V. (1988). *Lancet* **i**, 1059.
41. Josephs, S.F., Buchbinder, A., Streicher, H. *et al.* (1988). *Leukemia* **2**, 132–135.
42. Ablashi, D.V., Josephs, S.F., Buchbinder, A. *et al.* (1988). *J. Virol. Meth.* **21**, 29–48.
43. Jarrett, R.F., Gledhill, S., Qureshi, F. *et al.* (1988). *Leukemia* **2**, 496–502.
44. Krueger, G.R.F. (1988). *Lancet* **ii**, 518.
45. Biberfeld, P., Petren, A.-L., Eklund, A. *et al.* (1988). *J. Virol. Meth.* **21**, 49–60.
46. Eizuru, Y., Minematsu, T., Minamishima, Y. *et al.* (1989). *Lancet* **i**, 40.
47. Gendelman, H.E., Phelps, W., Feigenbaum, L. *et al.* (1986). *Proc. Natl Acad. Sci. USA* **83**, 9759–9763.
48. Nabel, G.J., Rice, S.A., Knipe, D.M. and Baltimore, D. (1988). *Science* **239**, 1299–1302.
49. Horvat, R.T., Wood, C. and Balachandran, N. (1989). *J. Virol.* **63**, 970–973.
50. Schnittman, S.M., Psallidopoulos, M.C., Clifford Lane, H. *et al.* (1989). *Science* **245**, 305–308.

51. Meyerhans, A., Cheynier, R., Albert, J. *et al.* (1989). *Cell* **58**, 901–910.
52. Fox, J., Briggs, M. and Tedder, R.S. (1988). *Lancet* **ii**, 396–397.
53. Webster, A., Cook, D.G., Emery, V.C. *et al.* (1989). *Lancet* **ii**, 63–66.
54. Browning, G.F. and Studdert, M.J. (1989). *Arch. Virol.* **104**, 77–86.
55. Kishi, M., Harada, H., Takahashi, M. *et al.* (1988). *J. Virol.* **62**, 4824–4827.
56. Efstathiou, S., Gompels, U.A., Craxton, M.A., Honess, R.W. and Ward, K. (1988). *Lancet* **i**, 63–64.
57. Lawrence, G.L., Chee, M., Craxton, M.A., Gompels, U.A., Honess, R.W. and Barrell, B.G. (1990). *J. Virol.* **64**, 287–299.
58. Honess, R.W., Gompels, U.A., Barrell, B.G. *et al.* (1989). *J. Gen. Virol.* **70**, 837–855.
59. Beck, S. and Barrell, B.G. (1988). *Nature, Lond.* **331**, 269–272.
60. Bapat, A.R., Bodner, A.J., Ting, R.C.Y. and Cheng, Y.-C. (1989). *J. Virol.* **63**, 1400–1403.
61. Agut, H., Collandre, H., Aubin, J.-T. *et al.* (1989). *Res. Virol.* **140**, 219–228.
62. Russler, S.K., Tapper, M.A. and Carrigan, D.R. (1989). *Lancet* **ii**, 382.

9 | New Hepatitis Agents

JOHN SALDANHA, JON MONJARDINO, MERON JACYNA,
PETER KARAYIANNIS and HOWARD THOMAS

*Department of Medicine, Queen Elizabeth the Queen Mother
Wing, St Mary's Hospital Medical School, London, W2 1NY, UK*

The hepatitis viruses are important human pathogens that cause both acute and chronic liver disease and in the case of hepatitis B virus hepatocellular carcinoma. The genomes of both hepatitis A and B viruses have been cloned and sequenced in recent years and their molecular biology extensively studied. In 1977 Rizzetto *et al.* [1] recognized and identified a new hepatitis agent, the delta virus, as a major factor influencing the severity of chronic hepatitis B infection. Isolation of the virus and successful cloning of the viral genome in several laboratories in recent years has enabled a detailed study of the structure and molecular biology of this viroid-like human hepatitis virus and of its biologically intriguing association with hepatitis B virus. These studies, as well as recently published advances on both parenterally and enterically transmitted non-A, non-B hepatitis, will be the subject of the present review.

9.1 DELTA VIRUS

9.1.1 Introduction

The discovery of the delta agent was reported in 1977 when Rizzetto and his collaborators decribed a new liver antigen, unrelated to HBV antigens, associated with chronic hepatitis B infection [1]. The agent behaves as a defective virus, requiring a helper function from HBV for propagation, and is coated in HBsAg. Infection with the delta agent occurs either at the same time as HBV (co-infection) or as super-infection in an established chronic HBV infection. In co-infection a self-limiting acute delta infection with clearance of both viruses is the most frequent outcome, although a higher incidence of fulminant hepatitis has been reported. Super-infection of the patients with chronic HBV infection on the other hand is frequently associated with persistent HDV infection

AIDS AND THE NEW VIRUSES
ISBN 0–12–200740–9

(70–90% of cases) and deterioration of the chronic hepatitis [2]. Delta virus super-infection does not appear to occur preferentially in any particular type of HBV chronic carrier: both HBeAg and anti-HBe carriers are susceptible [3]. Infection with hepatitis delta virus is associated with the detection of delta antigen and viral RNA in both liver and serum and with the development of antibodies to delta antigen (anti-HDV).

Serological findings distinguish acute from chronic HDV. The acute self-limiting disease is characterized by the presence of low titres of IgM and IgG anti-HDV. Following an early antigenaemic stage, the IgM antibody response usually lasts 2–3 weeks with IgG developing later. This pattern contrasts with chronic delta infection, arising from co- or super-infection where both IgM and IgG anti-HD persist throughout the disease [1]. HDV appears to have an inhibitory effect on the replication of HBV: most patients exhibit low levels of serum HBV DNA and are anti-HBe positive [4]. High levels of replication of both viruses have been described in some patients [5] and demonstrated within individual cells by double immunostaining with specific antibodies (R. Goldin, personal communication; [6]).

Experimental infection with HDV has been successfully achieved in those higher primates which can support productive HBV replication and recently also in the eastern woodchuck chronically infected with the HBV-related woodchuck hepatitis virus [7]. In both cases it has been shown that the progeny virions bear the coat of the co-infecting or already replicating virus, which in the case of the woodchuck results in a "new" WHVsAg coated HDV particle.

Transmission of HDV is, as with HBV, mainly by the parental route and associated with contact with blood or blood-derived products. Vertical transmission appears to be a rare event. Screening for HBsAg minimizes but does not abolish the risk of post-transfusion HDV hepatitis [8].

HDV infection has been reported world-wide and although its prevalence tends, in general, to correlate with the prevalence of HBV, it appears still not to have penetrated certain regions of high HBV endemicity including the Far East, Southern Africa and the Alaskan Eskimos. Striking differences in the prevalence of HDV to HBV infection have also been noted in neighbouring countries (Roumania vs. Bulgaria or Yugoslavia) [9, 10] or in different regions of one country (Kenya) [11], suggesting either an early stage of HDV dissemination or involvement of additional factors in the spread of the infection.

9.1.2 Structure and organization of the HDV genome

The virus particles are 35–37 nm in diameter (buoyant density 1.25 g/cm^3) [12] and are made up of a circular single-stranded RNA genome, about 1700 nucleotides long [13–18], associated with HDAg and encapsulated in HBV surface antigen (HBsAg). Unlike HBV, the RNA–HDAg complex does not form a nucleocapsid structure. HDV is the smallest known human virus and the first animal virus identified with a circular single-stranded RNA genome. Several groups have obtained cDNA clones covering part [13–15, 19, 20] or the whole of the genome [13, 14, 16]. The RNA used in these studies was obtained either from HDV isolated from the serum of a chronically infected chimpanzee [13, 15, 19], human serum [18, 20], or directly extracted from the liver of an infected woodchuck [16]. Studies show that the HDV genome undergoes extensive intramolecular base pairing to form an unbranched rod structure [13, 15]. Under non-denaturing conditions the RNA migrates as a 0.8 kbp fragment (Fig. 9.1), while denatured RNA has a mobility indicating a size of about 1.7 kbp (Fig. 9.2). Chimpanzee-derived HDV RNA is 1679 nucleotides long [13, 14], and passage of this through woodchucks showed only minor virus sequence changes (98.5% homology) with no insertions or deletions, indicating that no substantial genome alteration occurs on limited passage of the virus through a different host [16]. Up to 70% of the nucleotides are base paired and a further 6% can form G–U pairs [13, 16]. The complete human-derived HDV RNA sequence by Makino *et al.* [18], has 1683 nucleotides with 89% homology to the chimpanzee- or woodchuck-derived sequences. A partial human-derived HDV RNA sequence [20], 380 nucleotides long, has 93% homology with the complete human sequence by Makino *et al.* [18] and 83% homology with the chimpanzee-derived sequence, indicating the existence of different strains of HDV.

Hybridization analysis has shown that there is no detectable homology between HDV RNA and HBV DNA or nucleic acids from infectious non-A non-B patients [21]. HDV shares several common features with a group of plant pathogens, the viroids, virusoids and satellite viruses. Viroids are small, single-stranded circular RNAs about 250–400 nucleotides long, which are capable of self-replication but, unlike HDV, do not code for any protein [22]. Virusoids are similar to viroids in size and structure, but are encapsulated together with single-stranded plant RNA viruses. They do not replicate autonomously but may be required for viral infectivity. However, HDV RNA is much larger than viroid or virusoid RNA, encodes for at least one protein — HDAg — and is surrounded by a coat of HBsAg. In this respect, HDV resembles the satellite RNAs

(a) (b)

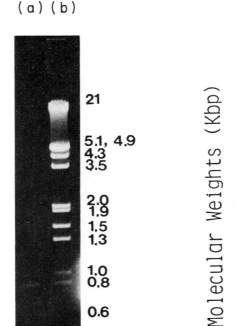

Fig. 9.1 Agarose gel analysis of native HDV RNA extracted from human serum. (a) HDV RNA; (b) λ-DNA fragments.

which are encapsulated in helper virus protein coats but are not capable of autonomous replication. The viroid consensus sequences GAAAC and GAUUUU which may be involved in viroid replication [23], are also present in the HDV genome. Throughout this review we use the numbering scheme of Wang *et al.* [13], which starts at a unique HindIII position. Note that this restriction site is missing in the other two complete sequences published. The sequence GAAAC is present twice (positions 88–92 and 940–944) in the chimpanzee-derived sequence [13], and in the human-derived sequence in different locations (positions 152–156 and 943–947) [18]. The sequence GAUUUU, on the other hand, is present once in the chimpanzee-derived genome (position 1453–1458) and again in a different location in the human-derived viral RNA (position 1479–1484). Conservation of the GAAAC sequence in the HDV isolates is suggestive of its possible involvement in HDV RNA replication.

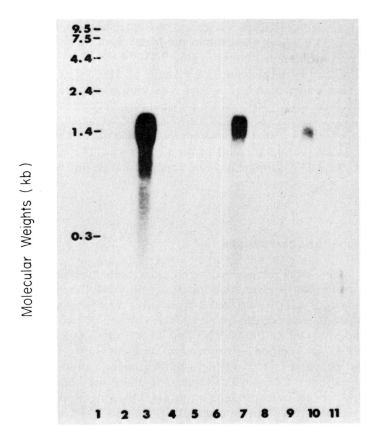

Fig. 9.2 Northern blot hybridization of denatured RNA extracted from sera with a ^{32}P-labelled HDV cDNA. Lanes 2, 4, 6 and 8, normal sera; lanes 3, 5, 7 and 10, HDV+ sera; lanes 1, 9 and 11, HBV+ sera.

Analysis of the HDV sequences has shown the presence of several open reading frames, both on the genomic and antigenomic strands. There are five potential open reading frames; two on the genomic strand and three on the antigenomic strand (the sequence of Kuo *et al.* [16] only has one of the antigenomic ORFs). The ORFs from the chimpanzee-derived sequences are similar and four of these are conserved in the human HDV isolate. The antigenomic ORF, starting at position 1619 (frame −2), has been shown to code for delta antigen. Fusion proteins expressed from this ORF are recognized by human anti-HDAg antibodies [13, 16, 24]. The size of the protein predicted from the RNA sequence varies amongst different isolates (Table 9.1).

Heterogeneity in the sequence of Wang *et al.* [13, 14] at position 1012 predicts two polypeptides, 214 and 195 amino acids long, with no significant homology with known polymerases or proteases [13]. The amino acid sequence is highly conserved between the human and chimpanzee isolates [18] and shows charged amino acids at the *N*-terminal end and uncharged amino acids at the *C*-terminus. The other predicted ORFs of the HDV genome do not appear to code for any functional protein.

9.1.3   Hepatitis delta antigen

Hepatitis delta virus antigen extracted from both liver and serum has been characterized in several laboratories with variable results. Western blot analysis of HDAg extracted from liver and serum of humans, chimpanzees or woodchucks shows either a single or two predominant polypeptides 27 000 or 29 000(P27) and 24 000 or 27 000 daltons (P24) [16, 24–30]. In addition, liver-derived antigen shows several lower molecular weight species thought to be degradation products. The two main polypeptides, P27 and P24, appear to share the same epitopes, as Western blot with different human anti-HDAg sera produce the same staining patterns [27]. Further analysis of P24 and P27 has been carried out by cloning part or the whole of the HDAg open reading frame in expression vectors [13, 16, 21, 24, 30]. Expression of the whole open reading frame from a chimpanzee-derived HDV clone in bacterial and yeast cells gave two proteins, 2400 and 2700 daltons, which were shown to be identical to the natural HDAg proteins P24 and P27, by Western blotting immunoabsorption experiments [29]. The authors suggested that heterogeneity in the open reading frame at position 1012, which introduced an amber stop codon in some clones, resulted in the two polypeptides which differed in their carboxyl termini. In contrast, Chang *et al.* [30] used human-derived HDV clones or RNA to express the HDAg gene. Expression of a plasmid containing the SV40 T antigen promotor and the HDAg gene in COS cells, or translation of antigenomic HDV RNA, transcribed from a cDNA clone, in rabbit reticulocyte lysates resulted in a single 2600 dalton polypeptide. In both cases the protein, which was phosphorylated but not glycosylated, was RNA

Table 9.1 Predicted open reading frame coding for HDAg using the published sequences.

Reference	Nucleotide positions of ORF	Total no. of amino acids	Nucleotide position of first AUG	Total no. of amino acids beginning with first AUG	Molecular weight of protein (daltons)
Wang *et al.* [13, 14]	1619–957/1014[a]	221/202[a]	1598	214/195[a]	24 000/22 000[a]
Kuo *et al.* [16, 17]	1619–1014	202	1598	195	22 000
Makino *et al.* [18]	1607–960	216	1601	214	24 000

[a] Ambiguity arising from clonal heterogeneity at nucleotide position 1012.

binding and located primarily in the cell nucleus. Other studies have also shown the accumulation of HDAg in the nuclei of infected cells by immunoperoxidase staining [24, 29, 31].

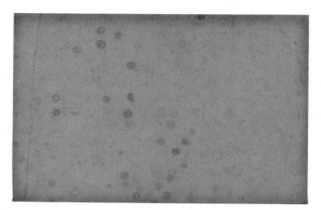

Fig. 9.3 Immunoperoxidase nuclear staining of a liver section from an HDV-infected woodchuck with rabbit antiserum raised against a fragment of the HDAg near the *N*-terminal end, showing nuclear staining.

Recent experiments suggest that HDAg epitopes reside at the *N*-terminal end of the protein between positions 1540–1364 (1366–1562, [24]; 1364–1540, [16]). Antibodies raised against a polypeptide ($D280_E$) expressed from this region of the genome gave patterns of staining of liver sections and immunoblots identical to those for anti-HDAg positive human serum [24] (Fig. 9.3). Complete inhibition of staining by anti-delta human serum of liver sections pre-incubated with the anti-$D280_E$ serum indicates that antibodies to all the HDAg epitopes are present in this serum. Comparison of the amino acid sequences of the published HDV sequences of this region show very few amino acid changes. It is likely that the two major polypeptides, P24 and P27 identified by some workers share the same epitopes, but the number of polypeptides making up the HDAg is still uncertain and will only be determined by amino acid sequencing of naturally-derived HDAg.

9.1.4 Replication strategy of the virus

The similarity between the structure of HDV RNA and viroids suggests that, as with viroids, replication occurs by a rolling circle mechanism [32]. In the original asymmetric model, a circular plus strand is copied to give a multimeric minus strand (Fig. 9.4(a)). In the alternative symmetric model, the multimeric minus strand is cleaved and circularized to give monomeric minus circles which are used as templates to generate multimeric, linear plus strands (Fig. 9.4(b)). Subsequent cleavage and circularization results in progeny viroid RNA molecules. Analysis of RNA species from infected livers (human, chimpanzee and woodchuck) support the symmetric rolling circle model of replication for HDV. Viral RNA species comprising linear genomic length RNA, circular genomic and antigenomic RNA species, as well as multimeric RNAs of both polarities [31, 33] were predominantly found in the nuclei. As many as 30 000 copies of genomic RNA, predominantly single-stranded, and 5–22 times less antigenomic RNA, mostly if not exclusively double-stranded, were found per cell [33]. Confirmation of the findings was reported by Taylor *et al.* [34] after growing HDV in primary woodchuck hepatocytes. No viral DNA intermediates have been detected in infected livers and no evidence has been found for reverse transcription activity. Although the major RNA species were not polyadenylated, a minor (about 1% of the HDV RNA) transcript of about 0.8 kbp with a poly A tail was sometimes observed, which may be the HDVAg mRNA [33].

It is clear from *in vivo* studies that HDV infection is dependent on prior infection or co-infection with HBV (in humans and chimpanzees) or WHV (in woodchucks). Although this suggests that the hepadnavirus surface antigen coating HDV particles may determine viral hepatropism, it remains unclear how HDV coated with human B surface antigen readily infects woodchuck hepatocytes, and an as yet unidentified delta specific gene product may be involved. Since progeny virus is encapsidated with hepadnavirus surface antigen, production of surface antigen is an essential requirement for delta virus multiplication. Establishment of an *in vitro* model for HDV infection [34, 35] has enabled an examination of the role of the helper hepadnavirus during HDV replication. This was achieved in monolayer cultures of primary hepatocytes from uninfected or chronically infected woodchucks, which were successfully infected with HDV. Only a small fraction of the cells supported virus replication, but the levels of viral RNA in these cells was comparable to those in liver cells infected *in vivo* and again it was predominantly detected in the nucleoplasm. However, in this system replication was incomplete and release of progeny virus was not demonstrated. Infection with HDV was successful both in the presence or absence of co-infection with WHV. Woodchuck hepatitis virus replication was never demonstrated *in vitro*, in cultures derived from infected hepatocytes or in cultures freshly infected, either in the presence or absence of HDV. These studies indicate that replication of a hepadnavirus is not a prerequisite for HDV replication.

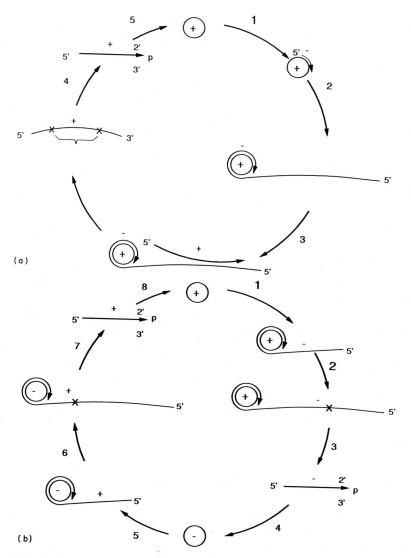

Fig. 9.4 Asymmetric (a) and symmetric (b) models of rolling-circle replication. The replication models begin at the top of each diagram, with an infecting circular plus strand (+) which becomes a template for minus-strand (−) synthesis (Step 1). In the asymmetric cycle a multimeric linear minus strand is copied into a multimeric plus-strand precursor (Step 3), and the plus-strand precursor is cleaved (Step 4) and circularized (Step 5). In the symmetric cycle, the multimeric minus strand is first cleaved to unit length (Step 3) and circularized (Step 4). The circular minus strand then serves as a rolling-circle template for the synthesis of a plus-strand precursor (Step 5), and this precursor is cleaved (Step 6) and ligated (Step 8).

In addition, Taylor *et al.* [34] have shown that primary hepatocyte cultures could only be infected with woodchuck-derived HDV; infection with virus from a human source was unsuccessful. In addition, neither primary duck hepatocytes nor two continuous human hepatoma cell lines, Hep G2 and Hep 3B, supported replication.

Further confirmation that hepadnavirus replication is unnecessary for HDV replication comes from studies by Gowans *et al.* [31], who used *in situ* hybridization to examine HDV and hepadnavirus markers in liver sections from infected animals. These authors reported that both HDV RNA and HDAg, located in the nuclei of hepatocytes with HDV RNA replication, were present in cells lacking markers of HBV replication. In persistently infected livers, single scattered cells containing both HDV RNA and Ag were found, in contrast to the focal distribution of the infected cells characteristic of HBV infection. Although replication of HDV RNA was closely associated with HDAg expression, some cells with replicating RNA were found to be HDAg negative.

Recently, Kuo *et al.* [36] demonstrated the replication of HDV RNA in monkey kidney (COS) and human hepatocellular carcinoma (HuH7) cell lines by transfection with an SV40-based eukaryotic expression vector containing three copies of the HDV genome. Both genomic and antigenomic RNA were detected in all transfected cell nuclei and HDAg accumulated in the nucleoli. Using an HDV sequence with a 2 base pair deletion in the HDAg open reading frame, these workers showed that HDAg is essential for HDV RNA replication and can act in "*trans*". Both the cellular location of HDAg and its postulated role in RNA replication are in conflict with previous reports which showed HDAg predominantly associated with the nucleoplasm [24, 29] and the presence of viral RNA in cells not displaying HDAg [31].

9.1.5 Processing of the RNA *in vivo* and *in vitro*

Present work has focused on the processing of HDV RNA during replication. In the rolling circle model of replication, cleavage of multimeric RNA followed by ligation is necessary to produce monomeric circles. Such cleavage and ligation reactions, which occur in the absence of protein, have been demonstrated in viroids, virusoids, plant satellite viruses and certain RNA sequences such as group I and II introns [37–40]. These self-cleaving RNAs, or ribozymes, require divalent cations and neutral or higher pH for self-cleavage to occur. Similar *in vitro* studies with transcribed delta RNA have shown that self-cleavage of antigenomic RNA occurs between nucleotides 900 and 901 [17, 41a, 42,

43], or between positions 685 and 686 of genomic RNA, and results in a 5' hydroxyl and 2'-3' monophosphate ends.

HDV RNA self-cleavage is much faster and dependent on a much lower Mg^{2+} concentration (10 mM Mg^{2+}) than other self-cleaved reactions [38]. The minimum flanking sequences required for efficient self-cleavage are 17 bases on the 5' side and 69 bases on the 3' side for antigenomic RNA, and 30 bases on the 5' side and 74 bases on the 3' side for genomic RNA. Unlike other self-cleaving RNAs, these sequences do not fit into a "hammerhead" structure [38, 44]. Longer HDV RNA subfragments are cleaved less efficiently, probably due to formation of secondary structure by intramolecular base pairing [17, 43].

Self-ligation of the fragments resulting from self-cleavage can occur on removal of Mg^{2+} ions [41b, 42]. However, only fragments with ligatable ends held in close proximity by intramolecular binding can re-ligate. Thus, during HDV RNA replication, the self-complementarity of the RNA would ensure that the two cleaved ends of linear monomeric RNA are brought into apposition and self-ligate.

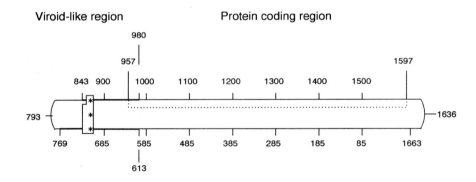

Fig. 9.5 Genomic map of the delta agent. The genomic RNA of the delta agent is drawn as a collapsed circle. A viroid-like domain at the left end of the molecule contains conserved segments (marked by heavy lines), the UV-sensitive element present in an RNase TI-resistant region (boxed and starred), and autocatalytic cleavage sites at residues 685 and 900. In the protein-coding region, the portion of the molecule specifying the delta antigen spans the distance between residues 957 and 1597 (designated by an open box); the actual mRNA for the antigen is composed of antigenomic sequences.

Based on the RNA structure, Branch *et al.* [45] have proposed that the HDV genome is made up of two domains; a small, highly conserved domain and a larger, less conserved domain which includes the HDAg gene (Fig. 9.5). The smaller domain (positions 613–980), which has no apparent coding capacity, has an ultraviolet-sensitive region which is highly conserved between the four reported HDV sequences, and is similar in size to viroids (250–400 nucleotides). In viroids, a UV-sensitive region in a highly conserved region of the genome is thought to be involved in replication. Branch *et al.* [45] speculate that HDV RNA may have originated from two different RNA molecules: a viroid-like free-living RNA associated with a messenger RNA.

9.1.6 Treatment of delta virus

Specific and sensitive hybridization-based assays for the detection of delta RNA, both in serum and liver, are now available [5, 46]. Although the presence of delta antigen in the liver by immunohistology remains the most sensitive marker of chronic infection, the non-invasive serum assays for viral RNA, which correlate well with intrahepatic HDAg, are preferred. Coupled with the existing commercial immunoassays for the detection of delta antigen and antibody, these newly developed molecular hybridization assays, particularly when using non-isotopic probes, will be invaluable for the further characterization of the disease, evaluation of infectivity, and monitoring of antiviral therapy. *Escherichia coli*-expressed delta antigens [24] and hyperimmune polyclonal antisera raised against them may soon replace current commercially produced human- or woodchuck-derived reagents, which are difficult to standardize, invariably contaminated with HBV antigens or antibodies, and a possible source of infection from other pathogens.

Several groups have shown that lymphoblastoid and recombinant α-interferon will inhibit HDV replication, at least for the duration of the therapy [47–49]. HDV RNA usually reappears in the serum within months following withdrawal of therapy. Trials of more protracted interferon therapy are now being undertaken.

9.2 PARENTERAL NON-A, NON-B HEPATITIS

Serological tests for the virus causing hepatitis B were developed in 1965 and for hepatitis A in 1973; it was then realized that many cases of post-transfusion hepatitis were not related to either of these agents, or to any other known viruses (Table 9.2) [50]. At this time, the term "non-A, non-B" hepatitis was first coined in an attempt to label this presumed hepatic infection.

Table 9.2   Incidence of post-transfusion hepatitis in various studies.

Reference	Number studied	Percentage developing hepatitis	Percentage due to:		
			HBV	NANB	Other
Prince et al. [94][a]	204	25	29	71	—
Alter et al. [95][a]	108	11	25	75	—
Knodell et al. [96][a]	279	17	6	88	6[b]
Seeff et al. [97]	2204	11	22	78	—
Alter et al. [98][a]	388	8	10	87	3[b]
Seeff et al. [99]	969	14	13	87	—
Aach et al. [100]	595	13	13	87	—
Tateda et al. [101[c]	1082	12	7	93	—
Dienstag et al. [102][d]	21	47	0	100	—
Papaevangelou [103][e]	250	7	17	78	5[b]
Nagatsuka et al. [104][a,b]	204	30	0	100	—

[a] Cardiovascular surgery patients.
[b] All CMV cases.
[c] Japanese study.
[d] Volunteers receiving malaria-rich blood.
[e] Thalassaemic children in Greece.

Identifying the agent responsible so that serological tests can be developed to screen blood and blood products for the presence of this agent is of prime importance, as non-A, non-B (NANB) hepatitis is a major cause of morbidity and mortality. Acute fulminant NANB hepatitis has a higher fatality rate than any other form of viral hepatitis [51] and it has also been estimated that between 40 and 50% of those acquiring NANB infection will develop chronic hepatitis, with 15–20% of these subjects progressing to cirrhosis [52]. For example, in the USA it has been estimated that approximately 6000 patients per annum develop cirrhosis as a direct consequence of chronic NANB hepatitis [53].

Over the past decade, much time and energy has been spent in trying to identify the agent(s) responsible for this disease, and now with the advances in molecular biology which have paralleled this period, an agent appears to have been isolated.

9.2.1 Nature of the agent

(a) Pathophysiology

Unlike hepatitis A and B infection, the NANB agent(s) are probably cytopathic, causing damage by direct lysis of hepatocytes [54]. In hepatitis A and B infection, there is immunologically mediated hepatocyte injury, both from the humoral and cellular arms of the immune system [55, 56]. In contrast, studies on hepatic autoreactivity in NANB infection indicate that it is unlikely that autoimmunity plays a significant role in mediating hepatocyte damage [57]. In support of this, histological studies have shown that there is in general a paucity of intrahepatic lymphocytes in NANB infection compared to hepatitis A and B infection [55]. Further support comes from studies on the effects of interferon treatment in chronic NANB hepatitis, where there is a fairly prompt fall in aminotransferase levels after interferon therapy is started [58]. This is in contrast to hepatitis B infection, where following initiation of therapy a rise in enzyme levels several weeks later indicates immune-mediated lysis of infected hepatocytes [59].

(b) How many agents

It is still not known whether NANB is caused by only one, or more than one agent. On the basis of physicochemical studies it has been suggested that there are probably two NANB agents; one that will pass through an 80-nm membrane filter, is sensitive to chloroform (indicating a lipid-containing envelope) and forms characteristic cytoplasmic tubules (HCV), and another agent which is resistant to chloroform and does not induce tubule formation [60]. Studies on the incubation periods of NANB hepatitis have also suggested that there may be two types, one with short (1–4 weeks) and a second with long (6–10 weeks) incubation periods [61]. Cross-challenge experiments in chimpanzees have shown that it is possible to sequentially infect animals with both of these agents, suggesting that these two agents are immunologically distinct [62]. Haemophiliacs are more likely to develop "short incubation" NANB hepatitis, suggesting that factor VIII concentrate is the carrier for this agent [63], whereas blood transfusion recipients are more likely to get "long-incubation" NANB, suggesting that whole blood is the source of this agent [50]. However, as both factor VIII and whole blood are derived from the same heterogeneous pool of donors, it is somewhat surprising that the short incubation agent should be associated solely with factor VIII. It may be that the short incubation period, rather than indicating a separate NANB agent, may instead be related to the recognized immunological abnormalities seen in many haemophiliacs [64], allowing the faster onset of hepatitis. Further support for a single-agent causing all types of NANB hepatitis comes from data showing that short incubation and long incubation disease can be caused in the same animal by increasing the dose of inoculum [65]. Thus, although there is evidence supporting both the single- and multiple-agent theories, on balance the data favour there being at least two agents.

9.2.2   Possible candidates

(a) *Retroviruses*

Much excitement occurred when reverse transcriptase activity was detected in some sera known to transmit NANB infection [66]. This strongly suggested that a retrovirus or retrovirus-like agent was the cause of the infection. Unfortunately, the promise of this early report was not fulfilled and several other groups have not been able to reproduce the results. Ultrastructural studies showing alterations in the cytoplasm of both hepatocytes and lymphocytes in chronic NANB hepatitis, which are similar to those found in other known retroviral infections, were initially interpreted as supporting the involvement of a retrovirus in NANB. More recent studies suggest that these changes may be caused by circulating interferon [67]. These results have, however, raised the possibility that the NANB agent may reside in peripheral blood lymphocytes, and indeed it has been shown that isolated, washed mononuclear cells from infected patients are infectious and transmit the disease [68].

(b) *Togaviruses*

Recent work has indicated that an RNA virus, which may be related to the togaviridae or flaviviridae families, is likely to be the cause of a large proportion of parenterally transmitted NANB hepatitis cases [69a, 69b]. Initial suspicion that a small, lipid enveloped RNA virus was responsible, came from studies by Bradley and colleagues in the USA who performed extensive physicochemical studies on the nature of the NANB agent. They found that it was sensitive to chloroform (indicating a lipid-containing envelope) and would pass through an 80-nm membrane filter

[70]. The togaviruses (which cause dengue, yellow fever and various types of encephalitis) are a group of small enveloped RNA viruses which have the same physicochemical properties as described and also induce similar cytoplasmic and ultrastructural changes [70]. Confirmation that an RNA virus is responsible has come from the Chiron Corporation in the USA, who recently have identified a cDNA clone from a random-primed cDNA library from infectious plasma [69b]. This clone is derived from an RNA virus and the authors indicate that it appears to be related to the togaviridae and to the flaviviridus genus. Using a yeast expression system to express viral protein from this cDNA clone has allowed the detection of antibody in the sera of patients with NANB hepatitis. Preliminary reports indicate that 70–80% of patients in the USA, Japan and Italy with chronic NANB hepatitis have antibodies to this virus [69a]. This antibody to the NANB agent (termed hepatitis C virus or HCV) unfortunately is only detectable in 15% of acute NANB infections, and this will be unlikely to help in the differential diagnosis of acute viral hepatitis. Nevertheless, it should prove extremely useful in patients with chronic NANB hepatitis. It seems likely that the remaining 20–30% of chronic NANB carriers have another as yet undiscovered virus.

9.2.3 Treatment

It is thought that α-interferon may be of value in the treatment of chronic NANB hepatitis. Two uncontrolled pilot studies in patients with chronic NANB infection have now been performed [58, 71] and have shown early encouraging results with aminotransferase levels returning to normal within 2 months of therapy in at least 80% of patients, and histological improvement being demonstrated in some subjects after a year's continuous therapy [58]. Controlled studies are now being performed in several centres and provisional results confirm the earlier findings of rapid normalization of aminotransferase levels in the majority of patients on low-dose α-interferon [72]. Of course the long-term goal is "cure", with normalization of aminotransferase levels and histology even after treatment has been discontinued. Preliminary results have suggested that, at least in some patients, one year's continuous therapy may be successful in bringing about a permanent biochemical and histological remission [58]. However, even if relapse occurs on stopping therapy, continuous low-dose interferon is reasonably well tolerated by patients and is an acceptable inconvenience in view of the high risk of development of cirrhosis.

9.3   ENTERICALLY TRANSMITTED NON-A, NON-B HEPATITIS

9.3.1   Epidemiology

Between December 1955 and January 1956 there were an estimated 29 000 icteric cases of hepatitis in New Delhi, India [73, 74], which occurred following large-scale contamination of the city's water supply system with sewage. The unimodal occurrence of the illness was indicative of transmission from a common source and the outbreak was initially attributed to infection with hepatitis A virus (HAV). However, serological testing for HAV markers in sera from 69 individuals revealed the presence of IgG and absence of IgM class antibodies, indicating prior immunity to the virus. Hepatitis B virus could only be implicated in seven of the cases [75, 76]. This new type of hepatitis has been termed enterically transmitted non-A, non-B (ET-NANB) hepatitis, emphasizing its water-borne, enteric route of transmission and setting it apart from the parenteral NANB virus(es).

There have been subsequent reports describing the occurrence of both epidemic and sporadic forms of ET-NANB hepatitis in India [77–79], Nepal [80], Burma [81], Pakistan [82] and the Tashkent region of the Soviet Union [83]. Outbreaks have also occurred in Algeria [84], Ivory Coast [85], Chad [86], Ghana [87], Somalia and Mexico. When such epidemics occur the characteristics of ET-NANB hepatitis make it easy to diagnose. However, hepatitis with characteristics similar to ET-NANB hepatitis occurs inbetween epidemics [79]. This sporadic or endemic form of ET-NANB hepatitis, if indeed it is due to ET-NANB hepatitis, is the most common cause of acute viral hepatitis in large parts of the developing world.

9.3.2   Disease characteristics

The incubation period of ET-NANB hepatitis ranges from 2–9 weeks with a mean of 6 weeks [73, 75, 76], the variability probably reflecting different virus dose or possibly involvement of different agents. The age distribution of disease during point-source epidemics seems to favour older individuals. In the New Delhi outbreak [73] the highest attack rate was in those aged 15–39 years, the prevalence of icteric disease being 1.3% in children under 15 years, 2.9% in young adults aged 15–39, and 2% in older age individuals. Similar findings have been reported by others [75, 77]. Higher attack rates with more uniform age distribution of disease have been observed under conditions of extreme overcrowding and poor sanitary conditions, such as the refugee camps of Africa.

In spite of high infection rates during epidemics, clinically apparent secondary cases are rare. This may suggest a high subclinical attack rate or poor person-to-person spread. In a study of household contacts of index cases of ET-NANB hepatitis abnormal liver function tests were found in about 20% of contacts. Since such abnormal liver function tests are found frequently in apparently healthy subjects, these findings should be viewed with caution.

Perhaps the most striking epidemiological feature of ET-NANB hepatitis is the high fatality rate associated with icteric disease. This stands at 1–2% of cases and is particularly high (10–20%) in women in the third trimester of pregnancy [75, 80]. Deaths are the result of fulminant hepatic failure.

Clinically ET-NANB hepatitis resembles HAV except for the high fatality rate, particularly in pregnancy. The disease is self-limiting and does not progress to chronicity. Apart from being jaundiced, more than 60% of the patients have anorexia and hepatomegaly, whilst fewer than 50% have fever, nausea, vomiting and pain [75, 76, 87].

The liver histology of patients with ET-NANB hepatitis appears to be characteristic of the condition and differs from the histopathological changes seen in hepatitis A and parenteral NANB. There is portal inflammation, large numbers of activated Kupffer cells and polymorphonuclear leukocytes but few lymphocytes, and hepatocytic and intracanalicular cholestasis have also been observed. Lobular scars with bridging and sub-massive hepatic necrosis have been seen in more severe cases [75].

9.3.3 Transmission studies

Balayan and co-workers [83] were the first to report transmission of ET-NANB hepatitis from a faecal extract of a human volunteer to two intravenously inoculated cynomolgus macaques. The animals developed alanine aminotransferase (ALT) elevations 24–36 days post-inoculation. Virus-like particles (VLPs) 27–30 nm in diameter were recovered from early phase stools (similar to those seen in the faecal extract from the human volunteer) [83]. African green monkeys were the next to be successfully infected with ET-NANB hepatitis, again using inocula positive for 27–30 nm VLPs [88]. Transmission of infection to tamarins has also been reported [80, 89, 90], but with varying success. Isocitrate dehydrogenase appears to be a better biochemical marker of liver dysfunction in these animals than ALT. Chimpanzees have also been infected [91].

The cynomolgus macaque (*Macaca fascicularis*) appears to be the best characterized animal model [80, 83, 89, 90]. Intravenous inoculation with faecal extracts results in disease in most of the animals injected, with ALT abnormalities occurring after a mean of 38 days post-inoculation [89, 90]. The histological evidence of the hepatitis consists of degeneration and necro-inflammatory changes in liver parenchyma, accompanied by inconspicuous or minimal infiltrations in portal tracts. Acidophilic degeneration and coagulative liver cell necrosis are also prominent. Serial passage of ET-NANB hepatitis in cynomolgus monkeys resulted in the shortening of the incubation period to 20 days, and if purified virus was used to a mean of 8 days [89, 90].

9.3.4   Virus characteristics

Recovery of VLPs from stools of humans and experimental animals with ET-NANB hepatitis was first reported by Balayan *et al.* [83]. VLPs 27–30 nm in diameter were detected in acute-phase stool from a human volunteer, and also from cynomolgus monkeys inoculated with this material. Similar size particles ranging from 27–34 nm in diameter have been reported by others [80, 82, 89–93]. Immune electron microscopy (IEM) has revealed the aggregation of these particles by acute and convalescent phase but not pre-inoculation sera. Virus is excreted prior to or during the initial increase in liver enzymes.

Morphologically many of the particles appear to have characteristic surface indentations and projections. Some particles lacking central cores display icosahedral symmetry, while others are partially disrupted [90].

Immune electron microscopy studies have revealed some puzzling features of the antibody response to the virus. Although both humans and experimental animals seroconvert after ET-NANB hepatitis infection, the antibody detected in acute phase serology is of higher titre than in convalescent sera. Moreover, the VLPs appear to be primarily coated by IgM class antibody [90]. Acute phase or convalescent sera from various outbreaks around the world have all been shown to aggregate a single proportion of ET-NANB hepatitis VLPs, suggesting that one virus or a serologically related class of viruses may be involved [92].

Attempts at purification of VLPs from stool preparations on CsCl gradients have shown that the virus is labile in dense salt solutions. The virus has a sedimentation coefficient of 183 S in linear, pre-formed sucrose gradients [90]. It is sensitive to freeze-thawing; particle counts decline in samples stored at $-20°C$ and immune aggregates degrade spontaneously when stored at 4–8°C. Virus capsid integrity is preserved by storage in liquid nitrogen and ions such as Mg^{2+} and Mn^{2+} may also be necessary to maintain structure. These physicochemical characteristics resemble those of the Norwalk virus [90].

Attempts to establish serological tests have been unsuccessful so far due to paucity of antigen and antibody. Such tests, further biochemical characterization and classification of the virus may have to await the cloning of the virus genome and expression of the virus capsid polypeptides.

9.4 CONCLUSION

As our knowledge of the structure and biology of the hepatitis viruses has increased and techniques for monitoring viral replication and level of viraemia have become available, attempts at therapy of the diseases caused by these agents have been made. Some success has already been achieved and further advances can be anticipated.

ACKNOWLEDGEMENTS

The authors thank Dr R. Goldin (Department of Histopathology, St Marys Hospital, London) for the photograph in Fig. 9.3 and Dr Branch for permission to reproduce Figs 9.4–9.6.

REFERENCES

1. Rizzetto, M., Canese, M.G., Arico, S. *et al.* (1977). Immunofluorescence detection of a new antigen-antibody system (delta/anti-delta) associated with the hepatitis B virus in the liver and in the serum of HBsAg carriers. *Gut* **18**, 997–1003.
2. Rizzetto, M. (1983). The delta agent. *Hepatology* **3**, 729–737.
3. Rizzetto, M., Ponzetto, A., Bonino, F. and Smedile, A. (1988). Hepatitis delta virus infection: clinical and epidemiological aspects. In *Viral Hepatitis and Liver Disease* (A. Zuckerman, ed.), pp. 389–394. Alan R. Liss, New York.
4. Moestrup, T., Hansson, B.G., Widell, A. and Nordenfelt, E. (1983). Clinical aspects of delta infection. *Br. Med. J.* (Clin. Res. Ed.) **286**, 87–90.
5. Saldanha, J., Di Blasi, F., Blas, C. *et al.* (1990). Detection of hepatitis delta virus RNA in chronic liver disease. *J. Hepatol.* **9**, 23–28.
6. Genesca, J., Jardi, R., Buti, M. *et al.* (1987). Hepatitis B virus replication in acute hepatitis B, hepatitis B virus, hepatitis delta virus coinfection and acute delta virus superinfection. *Hepatology* **7**, 569–572.

7. Ponzetto, A., Cote, P.J., Popper, H. *et al.* (1984). Transmission of the hepatitis B virus-associated agent to the eastern woodchuck. *Proc. Natl Acad. Sci. USA* **81**, 2208–2212.

8. Rosina, F., Saracco, G. and Rizzetto, M. (1985). Risk of post-transfusion infection with the hepatitis delta virus. *New Engl. J. Med.* **312**, 1488–1491.

9. Naoumov, N.W., Georgiev, A., Ognyanov, M. and Maleev, A. (1986). Infection with hepatitis delta virus in patients with fulminant hepatitis B and chronic HBsAg carriers in Bulgaria. *Hepato-Gastroenterol* **33**, 49–51.

10. Burek, V. (1987). Delta infection in Yugoslavia. In *The Hepatitis Delta Virus and its Infection* (M. Rizzetto, J. Gerin and R.H. Purcell, eds), Progress in Clinical and Biological Research, Vol. 234, p. 319. Alan R. Liss, New York.

11. Greenfield, C., Farci, P., Osidiana, V. *et al.* (1986). Hepatitis delta virus infection in Kenya. *Am. J. Epidemiol.* **123**, 416–423.

12. Bonino, F., Hoyer, B., Shih, J.W., Rizzetto, M., Purcell, R.H. and Gerin, J.L. (1984). Delta hepatitis agent: structural and antigenic properties of the delta-associated particle. *Infect. Immun.* **43**, 1000–1005.

13. Wang, K.-S., Choo, Q.-L., Weiner, A.J. *et al.* (1986). Structure, sequence and expression of the hepatitis delta (δ) viral genome. *Nature, Lond.* **323**, 508–514.

14. Wang, K.-S., Choo, Q.-L., Weiner, A.J. *et al.* (1987). Structure, sequence and expression of the hepatitis delta (δ) viral genome. *Nature, Lond.* **328**, 456.

15. Kos, A., Dijkema, R., Arnberg, A.C., van der Meide, P.H. and Schellekens, H. (1986). The hepatitis delta virus possess circular RNA. *Nature, Lond.* **323**, 558–560.

16. Kuo, M.Y.-P., Goldberg, J., Coates, L., Mason, W., Gerin, J. and Taylor, J. (1988). Molecular cloning of hepatitis delta virus RNA from an infected woodchuck liver: sequence, structure and application. *J. Virol.* **62**, 1855–1861.

17. Kuo, M.Y.-P., Sharmeen, L., Dinter-Gottlieb, G. and Taylor, J. (1988). Characterization of self-cleaving RNA sequences on the genome and antigenome of human hepatitis delta virus. *J. Virol.* **62**, 4439–4444.

18. Makino, S., Chang, M.-F., Shieh, C.-K. *et al.* (1987). Molecular cloning and sequencing of a human hepatitis delta virus RNA. *Nature, Lond.* **329**, 343–346.

19. Denniston, K.J., Hoyer, B.H., Smedile, A., Wells, F.V., Nelson, J. and Gerin, J.L. (1986). Cloned fragment of the hepatitis delta virus RNA genome: sequence and diagnostic application. *Science* **232**, 873–875.

20. Saldanha, J.A., Thomas, H.C. and Monjardino, J.P. (1987). Cloning and characterization of a delta virus cDNA sequence derived from a human source. *J. Med. Virol.* **22**, 323–331.

21. Weiner, A.J., Wang, K.-S., Choo, Q.-L., Gerin, J.L., Bradley, D.W. and Houghton, M. (1987). Hepatitis delta cDNA clones: undetectable hybridization to nucleic acids from infectious Non-A, Non-B hepatitis materials and hepatitis B DNA. *J. Med. Virol.* **21**, 239–247.

22. Riesner, D. and Gross, H.J. (1985). Viroids. *Ann. Rev. Biochem.* **54**, 531–564.

23. Diener, T.O. (1986). Viroid processing: A model involving the central conserved region and hairpin I. *Proc. Natl Acad. Sci. USA* **83**, 58–62.

24. Saldanha, J., Thomas, H.C. and Monjardino, J. (1988). Location of hepatitis delta virus antigen (HDVAg) epitope(s) within open reading frame 5 (ORF5). *1988 Meeting on Molecular Biology of Hepatitis B Viruses*. University of California, La Jolla, CA, p. 19.

25. Bonino, F., Heermann, K.H., Rizzetto, M. and Gerlich, W.H. (1986). Hepatitis delta virus: protein composition of delta antigen and its hepatitis B virus-derived envelope. *J. Virol.* **58**, 945–950.

26. Bergmann, K.F. and Gerin, J.L. (1986). Antigens of hepatitis delta virus in liver and serum of human and animals. *J. Infect. Dis.* **154**, 702–706.

27. Zyzik, E., Ponzetto, A., Forzani, B., Hele, C., Heermann, K.-H. and Gerlich, W.H. (1987). Viruses proteins of hepatitis delta virus in serum and liver. In *Hepadna Viruses*, p. 565–577. Alan R. Liss, New York.

28. Pohl, C., Baroudy, B.M., Bergmann, K.F. *et al.* (1987). A human monoclonal antibody that recognizes viral polypeptides and *in vitro* translation products of the genome of the hepatitis D virus. *J. Infect. Dis.* **156**, 622–629.

29. Weiner, A.J., Choo, Q.-L., Wang, K.-S. *et al.* (1988). A single antigenomic open reading frame of the hepatitis delta virus encodes the epitope(s) of both hepatitis delta antigen polypeptides p24 and p27. *J. Virol.* **62**, 594–599.

30. Chang, M., Baker, S.C., Soe, L.H. *et al.* (1988). Human hepatitis delta antigen is a nuclear phosphoprotein with RNA-binding activity. *J. Virol.* **62**, 2403–2410.

31. Gowans, E.J. Baroudy, B.M., Negro, F., Ponzetto, A., Purcell, R.H. and Gerin, J.L. (1988). Evidence for replication of hepatitis delta virus RNA in hepatocyte nuclei after *in vivo* infection. *Virology* **167**, 274–278.

32. Branch, A.D. and Robertson, H.D. (1984). A replication cycle for viroids and small infectious RNAs. *Science* **223**, 450–455.

33. Chen, P., Kalpana, G.M., Goldberg, J. *et al.* (1986). Structure and replication of the genome of the hepatitis delta virus. *Proc. Natl Acad. Sci. USA* **83**, 8774–8778.

34. Taylor, J., Mason, W., Summers, J. *et al.* (1987). Replication of human hepatitis delta virus in primary cultures of woodchuck hepatocytes. *J. Virol.* **61**, 2891–2895.

35. Choi, S.-S., Rasshofer, R. and Roggendorf, M. (1988). Propagation of woodchuck hepatitis delta virus in primary woodchuck hepatocytes. *Virology* **167**, 451–457.

36. Kuo, M.Y.-P., Chao, M. and Taylor, J. (1989). Initiation of replication of the human hepatitis delta virus genome from cloned DNA – role of delta antigen. *J. Virol.* **63**, 1945–1950.

37. Zang, A.J., Crabowski, P.J. and Cech, T.R. (1983). Autocatalytic cyclisation of an excised intervening sequence RNA is a cleavage-ligation reaction. *Nature, Lond.* **301**, 578–583.

38. Buzayan, J.M., Gerlach, W.L. and Bruening, G. (1986). Non-enzymatic cleavage and ligation of RNAs complementary to a plant virus satellite RNA. *Nature, Lond.* **323**, 349–353.

39. Forster, A.J. and Symonds, R.H. (1987). Self-cleavage of plus and minus RNAs of a viroid and a structural model for active sites. *Cell* **49**, 211–220.

40. Haseloff, J. and Gerlach, W.L. (1988). Simple RNA enzymes with new and highly specific endoribonuclease activities. *Nature, Lond.* **334**, 585–591.

41a. Sharmeen, L., Kuo, M.Y.-P., Dinter-Gottlieb, G. and Taylor, J. (1988).

Antigenomic RNA of human hepatitis delta virus can undergo self-cleavage. *J. Virol.* **62**, 2674–2679.

41b. Sharmeen, L., Kuo, M.Y.-P. and Taylor, J. (1989). Self-ligating RNA sequences on the antigenome of human hepatitis delta virus. *J. Virol.* **63**, 1428–1430.

42. Wu, H.-N. and Lai, M.M.C. (1989). Reversible cleavage and ligation of hepatitis delta virus RNA. *Science* **243**, 652–654.

43. Wu, H.-N., Lin, Y.-J., Lin, F.-P., Makino, S., Chang, M.-F. and Lai, M.M.C. (1989). Human hepatitis virus RNA subfragments contain an autocleavage activity. *Proc. Natl Acad. Sci. USA* **86**, 1831–1835.

44. Forster, A.C., Davies, C., Sheldon, C.C., Jeffries, A.C. and Symons, H. (1988). Self-cleaving viriod and newt RNAs may only be active as dimers. *Nature, Lond.* **334**, 265–267.

45. Branch, A.D., Benenfeld, B.J., Baroudy, B.M., Wells, F.V., Gerin, J.L. and Robertson, H.D. (1989). An ultraviolet sensitive RNA structural element in a viroid-like domain of the hepatitis delta virus. *Science* **243**, 649–652.

46. Smedile, A., Rizzetto, M., Denniston, K. *et al.* (1986). Type D hepatitis: the clinical significance of hepatitis D virus RNA in serum as detected by a hybridisation-based assay. *Hepatology* **6**, 1297–1302.

47. Hoofnagle, J., Mullen, K., Peters, M. *et al.* (1987). Treatment of chronic delta hepatitis with recombinant human alpha interferon. In *Hepatitis Delta Virus and its Infection*, p. 291–298. Alan R. Liss, New York.

48. Rosina, F., Saracco, G., Lattore, V. *et al.* (1987). Alpha 2 interferon in the treatment of chronic delta virus (HDV) hepatitis. In *Hepatitis Delta Virus and its Infection*, p. 299–303. Alan R. Liss, New York.

49. Thomas, H.C., Farci, P., Shari, R., Karayiannis, P., Smedile, A. and Gerin, C.L. (1987). Inhibition of hepatitis delta virus replication by lymphoblastoid human alpha interferon. In *Hepatitis Delta Virus and its Infection*, p. 277. Alan R. Liss, New York.

50. Feinstone, S.M., Kapikian, A.Z., Purcell, R.H., Alter, H.J. and Holland, P.V. (1975). Transfusion-associated hepatitis not due to viral hepatitis A or B. *New Engl. J. Med.* **292**, 767–770.

51. Mathieson, L.R., Skinhoj, P., Nielson, J.O., Purcell, R.H., Wong, D.C. and Ranek, L. (1980). Hepatitis A, B and Non-A, Non-B in fulminant hepatitis. *Gut* **23**, 270–275.

52. Realdi, G., Alberti, A., Rugge, M. *et al.* (1982). Long term follow up of acute and chronic Non-A, Non-B post-transfusion hepatitis; evidence of progression to liver cirrhosis. *Gut* **23**, 270–275.

53. Halliday, C. and Henahan, J. (1986). Congress Report; 1986 World Congress of Gastroenterology. *Gastroenterology in Practice* **2**, 6–16.

54. Dienes, H.P., Popper, H., Arnold, W. and Lobeck, H. (1982). Histologic observations in human hepatitis Non-A, Non-B. *Hepatology* **2**, 562–571.

55. Dienstag, J.L., Bhan, A.K., Klingenstein, R.J. and Svarese, A.M. (1982). Immunopathogenesis of liver disease associated with hepatitis B. In *Viral Hepatitis* (W. Szmuness, H.J. Alter and J.E. Maynard, eds), p. 221–236. Franklin Institute Press, Philadelphia.

56. Vallbracht, A., Gabriel, P., Maier, K. *et al.* (1986). Cell-mediated cytotoxicity in hepatitis A virus infection. *Hepatology* **6**, 1308–1314.

57. Vento, S., McFarlane, B.M., McSorley, C.G. *et al.* (1988). Liver

autoreactivity in acute virus A, B and Non-A, Non-B hepatitis. *J. Clin. Lab. Immunol.* **25**, 1–7.

58. Hoofnagle, J.H., Mullen, K.D., Jones, D.B. *et al.* (1986). Treatment of chronic Non-A, Non-B hepatitis with recombinant human alpha-interferon. *New Engl. J. Med.* **315**, 1575–1578.

59. Lok, A.S.F., Weller, I.V.D., Karayiannis, P. *et al.* (1984). Thrice weekly lymphoblastoid interferon is effective in inhibiting hepatitis B virus replication. *Liver* **4**, 45–49.

60. Bradley, D.W. (1985). The agents of Non-A, Non-B hepatitis. *J. Virol. Meth.* **10**, 307–319.

61. Dienstag, J.L. (1983). Non-A, Non-B hepatitis. In *Recent Advances in Hepatology*, Vol. 1 (H.C. Thomas and R.N.M. MacSween, eds), p. 25. Churchill Livingstone, Edinburgh.

62. Bradley, D.W., Maynard, J.E., Cook, E.H. *et al.* (1980). Non-A, Non-B hepatitis in experimentally infected chimpanzees; cross-challenge and electron microscopic studies. *J. Med. Virol.* **6**, 185–201.

63. Bamber, M., Murray, A., Arborgh, B.A.M. *et al.* (1980). Short incubation Non-A, Non-B hepatitis transmitted by factor VIII concentrates in patients with congenital coagulation disorders. *Gut* **22**, 854–859.

64. Froebel, K.S., Madhok, R., Forbes, C.D., Lennie, S.E., Lowe, G.D.O. and Sturrock, R.D. (1983). Immunological abnormalities in haemophilia; are they caused by American factor VIII concentrate? *Br. Med. J.* **287**, 1091–1093.

65. Brotman, B., Prince, A.M. and Huima, T. (1985). Is there more than one Non-A, Non-B agent? *J. Infect. Dis.* **151**, 618–623.

66. Seto, B., Coleman, W.G., Iwarson, S. and Geretry, R.J. (1984). Detection of reverse transcriptase activity in association with the Non-A, Non-B agent(s). *Lancet* **ii**, 941–943.

67. Schaff, Z., Gerety, R.J., Grimley, P.M. Iwarson, S.A., Jackson, D.R. and Tabor, E. (1985). Ultrastructural and cytochemical study of hepatocytes and lymphocytes during experimental Non-A, Non-B infections in chimpanzees. *J. Exp. Pathol.* **2**, 25–36.

68. Hellings, J.A., Van der veen-du Prie, J., Snelting-van Densen, R. and Stute, R. (1985). Preliminary results of transmission experiments of Non-A, Non-B hepatitis by mononuclear leucocytes from a chronic patient. *J. Virol. Meth.* **10**, 321–326.

69a. Kuo, M.Y.-P., Choo, Q.-L., Alter, H.J. *et al.* (1989). An assay for circulating antibodies to a major aetiologic virus of human Non-A, Non-B hepatitis. *Science* **244**, 362–364.

69b. Choo, Q.L., Kuo, G., Weiver, A.J., Overby, L.R., Bradley, D.W. and Houghton, M. (1989). Isolation of a cDNA clone derived from a blood-borne Non-A, Non-B viral hepatitis genome. *Science* **224**, 359–362.

70. Bradley, D.W., McCaustland, K.A., Cook, E.H., Schable, C.A., Ebert, J.W. and Maynard, J.E. (1985). Post-transfusion Non-A, Non-B hepatitis in chimpanzees; evidence that the tubule forming agent is a small enveloped virus. *Gastroenterology* **88**, 773–779.

71. Thomson, B.J., Doran, M., Lever, A.M.L. and Webster, A.D.B. (1987). Alpha-interferon therapy for Non-A, Non-B hepatitis transmitted by gammaglobulin replacement therapy. *Lancet* **i**, 539–541.

72. Jacyna, M.R., Brooks, G., Loke, R.H.T., Crossey, M., Murray-Lyon, I.M.

and Thomas, H.C. (1989). A controlled study of lymphoblastoid interferon in chronic Non-A, Non-B hepatitis; short term results. *Br. Med. J.* **298**, 80–82.

73. Viswanathan, R. (1957). Infectious hepatitis in Delhi (1955–56): a critical study, epidemiology. *Indian J. Med. Res.* (Suppl.) **45**, 1–30.

74. Naidu, S.S. and Viswanathan, R. (1957). Infectious hepatitis in Delhi (1955–56): a critical study, observations in pregnant women. *Indian J. Med. Res.* (Suppl.) **45**, 1–76.

75. Khuroo, M.S. (1980). Study of an epidemic of Non-A, Non-B hepatitis: possibility of another human hepatitis virus distinct from post-transfusion Non-A, Non-B type. *Am. J. Med.* **68**, 818–824.

76. Wong, D.C., Purell, R.H., Sreenivasan, M.A., Prasad, S.R. and Pavri, K.M. (1980). Epidemic and endemic hepatitis in India: evidence for a Non-A, Non-B hepatitis virus aetiology. *Lancet* **ii**, 876–879.

77. Sreenivasan, M.A., Banerjee, K., Pandya, P.G. *et al.* (1978). Epidemiological investigations of an outbreak of infectious hepatitis in Ahmedabad City during 1976. *Indian J. Med. Res.* **67**, 197–206.

78. Tandon, B.N., Joshi, Y.K., Jain, S.K., Gandhi, B.M., Mathiesen, L.R. and Tandon, H.D. (1982). An epidemic of Non-A, Non-B hepatitis in North India. *Indian J. Med. Res.* **75**, 739–744.

79. Khuroo, M.S., Duermeyer, W., Zargar, S.A., Ahanger, M.A. and Shah, M.A. (1983). Acute sporadic Non-A, Non-B hepatitis in India. *Am. J. Epidemiol.* **118**, 360–364.

80. Kane, M.A., Bradley, D.W., Shrestha, S.M. *et al.* (1984). Epidemic Non-A, Non-B hepatitis in Nepal. Recovery of a possible aetiologic agent and transmission studies in marmosets. *J. Am. Med. Assoc.* **252**, 3140–3145.

81. Myint, H., Soe, M.M., Khin, T., Myint, T.H. and Tin, K.M. (1985). A clinical and epidemiological study of an epidemic of Non-A, Non-B hepatitis in Rangoon. *Am. J. Trop. Med. Hygiene* **34**, 1183–1189.

82. De Cock, K.M., Bradley, D.W., Sandford, N.L., Govindarajan, S., Maynard, J.E. and Redeker, A.G. (1987). Epidemic Non-A, Non-B hepatitis in patients from Pakistan. *Ann. Intern. Med.* **106**, 227–230.

83. Balayan, M.S., Andjaparidze, A.G., Savinskaya, S.S. *et al.* (1983). Evidence for a virus in Non-A, Non-B hepatitis transmitted via the faecal–oral route. *Intervirology* **20**, 23–31.

84. Bellabes, H., Bourguermouh, A., Benatallah, A. and Illoul, G. (1985). Epidemic Non-A, Non-B viral hepatitis in Algeria: strong evidence for its spreading by water. *J. Med. Virol.* **16**, 257–263.

85. Sarthou, J.L., Budkowsk, A., Sharma, M.D., Lhuillier, M. and Pillot, J. (1986). Characterisation of an antigen–antibody system associated with epidemic Non-A, Non-B hepatitis in West Africa and experimental transmission of an infectious agent to primates. *Ann. Inst. Pasteur* **137E**, 225–232.

86. Molinie, C., Saliou, P., Roue, R. *et al.* (1988). Acute epidemic Non-A, Non-B hepatitis: a clinical study of 38 cases in Chad. In *Viral Hepatitis and Liver Disease* (A.J. Zuckerman, ed.), p. 154–157. Alan R. Liss, New York.

87. Morrow, R.H., Smetana, H.F., Sai, F.T. and Edgcomb, J.H. (1968). Unusual features of viral hepatitis in Accra, Ghana. *Ann. Intern. Med.* **68**, 1250.

88. Andjaparidze, A.G., Balayan, M.S., Saninov, A.P., Braginsky, D.M., Poleschuk, V.F. and Lamyatina, N.A. (1986). Faecal-orally transmitted Non-A, Non-B hepatitis induced in monkeys. *Vopr. Virus* **1**, 73–80.
89. Bradley, D.W., Krawczynski, K., Cook, E.H. *et al.* (1987). Enterically transmitted Non-A, Non-B hepatitis: serial passage of disease in cynomolgus macaques and tamarins and recovery of disease associated 27- to 34-nm virus like particles. *Proc. Natl Acad. Sci. USA* **84**, 6277–6281.
90. Bradley, D.W., Krawcynski, K., Cook, E.H. *et al.* (1988). Enterically transmitted Non-A, Non-B hepatitis: aetiology of disease and laboratory studies in non-human primates. In *Viral Hepatitis and Liver Disease* (A.J. Zuckerman, ed.), p. 138–147. Alan R. Liss, New York.
91. Arankalle, V.A., Ticehurst, J., Sreenivasan, M.A. *et al.* (1988). Aetiological association of a virus-like particle with enterically transmitted Non-A, Non-B hepatitis. *Lancet* **i**, 550–554.
92. Bradley, D.W., Andjaparidze, A., Cook, E.H. *et al.* (1988). Aetiological agent of enterically transmitted Non-A, Non-B hepatitis. *J. Gen. Virol.* **69**, 731–738.
93. Sreenivasan, M.A., Arankalle, V.A., Sehgal, A. and Pavri, K.M. (1984). Non-A, Non-B epidemic hepatitis: visualisation of virus-like particles in the stool by immune electron microscopy. *J. Gen. Virol.* **65**, 1005–1007.
94. Prince, A.H., Brotman, B., Grady, G.P. *et al.* (1984). Long-incubation post-transfusion hepatitis without serological evidence of exposure to hepatitis B virus. *Lancet* **ii**, 241–246.
95. Alter, H.J., Purcell, R.H., Holland, P.V., Feinstone, S.M., Morrow, A.G. and Moritsugu, Y. (1975). Clinical and serological analysis of transfusion-associated hepatitis. *Lancet* **ii**, 838–841.
96. Knodell, R.C., Conrad, M.E., Ginsberg, A.L. and Bell, C.J. (1976). Efficacy of prophylactic gamma globulin in preventing Non-A, Non-B post-transfusion hepatitis. *Lancet* **i**, 557–561.
97. Seeff, L.B., Zimmerman, H.J., Wright, E.C. *et al.* (1977). A randomised, double blind controlled trial of the efficacy of immune serum globulin for the prevention of post-transfusion hepatitis: a Veterans Administration cooperative study. *Gastroenterology* **72**, 111–121.
98. Alter, H.J., Purcell, R.H., Feinstone, S.M., Holland, P.V. and Morrow, A.G. (1978). Non-A, Non-B hepatitis: a review and interim report of an ongoing prospective study. In *Viral Hepatitis* (G.N. Vyas, S.N. Cohen and R. Schmid, eds), p. 359–369. Franklin Institute Press, Philadelphia.
99. Seeff, L.B., Wright, E.C., Zimmerman, H.J. *et al.* (1978). Post-transfusion hepatitis, 1973–1975: a veterans cooperative study. In *Viral Hepatitis* (G.N. Vyas, S.N. Cohen and R. Schmid, eds), p. 371–387. Franklin Institute Press, Philadelphia.
100. Aach, R.D., Lander, J.J., Sherman, L.A. *et al.* (1978). Transfusion-transmitted viruses: interim analysis of hepatitis among transfused and non-transfused patients. In *Viral Hepatitis* (G.N. Vyas, S.N. Cohen and R. Schmid, eds), p. 383–396. Franklin Institute Press, Philadelphia.
101. Tateda, A., KiKuchi, K., Numazaki, Y., Shirachi, R. and Ishido, N. (1979). Non-B hepatitis in Japanese recipients of blood transfusions: clinical and serologic studies after the introduction of laboratory screening of donor blood hepatitis B surface antigen. *J. Infect. Dis.* **139**, 511.
102. Dienstag, J.L., Krotoski, W.A., Howard, W.A. *et al.* (1981). Non-A, Non-

B hepatitis after experimental transmission of malaria by inoculation of blood. *J. Infect. Dis.* **143**, 200–209.

103. Papaevangelou, G. (1981). Non-A, Non-B hepatitis in Greece. In *Non-A, Non-B Hepatitis* (R.J. Gerety, ed.), p. 167–174. Academic Press, New York.

104. Nagatsuka, Y., Ohori, H., Kanno, A., Abe, Y., Togoh, T. and Ishida, N. (1983). A risk index for the prediction of the incidence of Non-A, Non-B post-transfusion hepatitis in open heart surgery patients. *J. Med. Virol.* **12**, 81.

Index

213